Private Practice Made Simple

Everything You Need to Know to Set Up and Manage a Successful Mental Health Practice

RANDY J. PATERSON, PhD

New Harbinger Publications, Inc.

Publisher's Note

This publication is designed to provide accurate and authoritative information in regard to the subject matter covered. It is sold with the understanding that the publisher is not engaged in rendering psychological, financial, legal, or other professional services. If expert assistance or counseling is needed, the services of a competent professional should be sought.

Distributed in Canada by Raincoast Books

Copyright © 2011 by Randy J. Paterson
            New Harbinger Publications, Inc.
            5674 Shattuck Avenue
            Oakland, CA 94609
            www.newharbinger.com

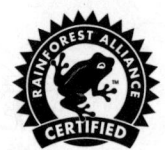

Cover design by Amy Shoup
Acquired by Melissa Kirk
Edited by Nelda Street

All Rights Reserved

Printed in the United States of America

Library of Congress Cataloging-in-Publication Data

Paterson, Randy J.
  Private practice made simple : everything you need to know to set up and manage a successful mental health practice / Randy J. Paterson.
     p. cm.
  Includes bibliographical references.
  ISBN 978-1-60882-023-8 (pbk.) -- ISBN 978-1-60882-024-5 (pdf ebook)
  1. Mental health counseling--Practice. 2. Psychotherapy--Practice. I. Title.
  RC466.P38 2011
  616.89'14--dc22

13   12   11

10   9   8   7   6   5   4   3   2   1

First printing

For Geoff

Contents

Acknowledgments vii

Introduction 1

CHAPTER 1
Why/Why Not: The Decision to Open a Practice . .5

CHAPTER 2
Who/Where: Names and Location 29

CHAPTER 3
Setting the Scene: The Office as Stage 53

CHAPTER 4
Getting Referrals. 75

CHAPTER 5
Creating a Website. 95

CHAPTER 6
Managing Client Information. 113

CHAPTER 7
Managing Finances 137

CHAPTER 8
The Clinic Assistant 161

CHAPTER 9
Managing Clinical Services 179

CHAPTER 10
The Ritual Clinic: Keeping Your Work
Sustainable 199

CHAPTER 11
The Long View: Burnout and Beyond. 223

Postscript 249

References 253

Index. 259

Acknowledgments

No one learns entirely by trial and error. While setting up my clinic and, much later, writing this book, I consulted more people than I can name. I am particularly grateful to the following friends and clinicians for their invaluable input: Dan Bilsker, Martha Capreol, Anne Howson, William Koch, Susan Mackey-Jamieson, Lisa Shatford, and Adrienne Wang. I am indirectly indebted to Richard Wright for the sailing metaphors and for making a bet that he would finish his book before I finished this one. He won.

Many thanks go to Barbara Fredrickson, who took time from her schedule to provide useful input that found its way into chapter 8. Paul Belserene broke me of the habit of writing rapid replies to e-mail, and he provided feedback on the original title of the book. Alain de Botton inspired me through his writing, and he pointed the way toward a useful quote. David Burns provided comments on passages involving clients' commitment to therapy. Marilyn Ransby offered useful clarification on some of the vagaries of U.S. taxes and health insurance. My early mentors Bill Newby, Jack Sweetland, and

Jim Neufeld provided many ideas that have survived the years and have found their way into this book.

I would also like to thank participants in the British Columbia Psychological Association Internet forum, who weighed in on issues including the attractions and anxieties of private practice, the dress of psychologists, and personal strategies for avoiding burnout. Those who provided suggestions include Galia Artzy, Robinder Bedi, Catherine Bond, Dianne Chappell, Elsie de Vita, Anne Dietrich, Cam Ellison, Jane Flint, Lynda Grant, Tracy Halpen, Amy Janeck, Peter Johnson, Gary Lea, Jeanne LeBlanc, Joanne MacKinnon, Rachel Mallory, Catherine McLaughlin, Alison Miller, Lynda Murdoch, Rami Nader, Theresa Nicassio, Serena Patterson, Don Ramer, Lara Robinson, Joti Samra, Susanne Schibler, Eroca Shaler, Raymond Shred, Charlotte Sutker, Maria Undurraga, John Wagner, Judy Weiser, and Alina Wydra.

I have offered workshops on practice management for several years and have shamelessly mined attendees' comments and observations for material for this book. To all such workshop participants, I give my thanks.

As always, the staff at New Harbinger Publications has been extremely encouraging and helpful. Matthew McKay is surely one of the most accessible and enthusiastic publishers in the business. Melissa Kirk guided the book from a flurry of acceptance e-mails to publication. Nelda Street provided detailed copyediting that markedly improved the tone and flow of the book. Regrettably, I can blame none of them for any failings, inaccuracies, or deficiencies, which are entirely my own contribution.

Geoff Bannoff provided useful input on financial concerns, website design, and computer security, based on his experience managing a much larger organization than most psychologists will ever have to face. His patience and endless support are most appreciated.

Introduction

Here's the big secret: No one really teaches you how to manage a mental health or counseling practice. As clinicians we stumble through our careers, gradually picking up shortcuts and strategies that make our lives (or those of our clients) a lot easier. Many of these useful ideas aren't rocket science and could have been taught to us in an afternoon if anyone had thought about it. That's what this book is for: it's nothing more than a collection of useful basic tips.

I attended a graduate program in clinical psychology that was aggressively research oriented. The course work emphasized research strategies. When treatment came up, it was in the form of outcome trials. We would learn all the details of the study design, the treatments applied (or not) to various groups of subjects, and the results obtained. We spent hours analyzing the type 1 error rate (per contrast, per time, per study?). Only two things were missed:

- How to conduct treatment
- How to practice in the field we were there to learn

Trivial, really.

I once walked unnoticed behind two faculty members who were discussing one of the perennial complaints of students: that our clinical psychology program wasn't training us to be clinical psychologists. "It's ridiculous," said one. "They can learn that in their spare time." The other nodded vigorously in agreement. The faint clattering sounds behind them were the scales falling from my eyes.

Our program did have one nod to clinical practice. It was called the "Proseminar in Clinical Psychology," and it was obvious that no one knew what it should be about. Bewildered adjunct faculty members were hauled in to brief the students on the world beyond the university gates. They talked about the client populations they saw, the tests they used, and the structure of their facilities' psychology departments—and then glanced nervously over at the instructor, who would shrug and smile.

We loved that class. It always ended early and, given that it was scheduled for midafternoon, allowed the clinical students to flee the building for the graduate student pub and get to know one another. Several marriages and quite a number of more temporary arrangements were attributable to those late afternoons at The Grad. But I don't think we learned much about running a practice.

When, after many years in hospital settings, I cut the apron strings and set out on my own, I quickly discovered the gaps in my training. I made mistake after mistake and began collecting advice from others. Even when I worked in institutional settings, my practice had always included teaching, and I eventually began offering professional workshops on private-practice management. I collected more ideas from my attendees. This book is the result.

The emphasis of the book is on quick and easy strategies that can save a lot of headaches. To supplement the contents, a set of additional downloadable forms and sample sheets is available at no charge online at my clinic's website, www.changeways.com, and at www.20238.nhpubs.com. I suggest that you take a minute to visit either site now and bookmark it or write down the URL and keep it handy for future reference.

A note on style: When training or supervising practitioners, I have often said that it is possible to treat a problem seriously without coming across like a funeral director. Indeed, some of the best interventions—even with clients suffering from depression, bereavement, or life-threatening illness—are those conducted with humor and a light touch. The same can be said for writings on the potentially arid topic of practice management. Although we might be tempted to take our work very seriously, within these pages let's try to relax, sit back, unclench, and remove the gowns of formality to which too many of us have become accustomed.

CHAPTER 1

Why/Why Not: The Decision to Open a Practice

I usually start my private practice workshops with a brief brainstorming session in which participants identify considerations that attract them to private practice and ones that make them want to run the other way. If they have already opened a practice despite their misgivings, I ask whether their hopes panned out and their fears proved justified. Here are the resulting top-ten lists: the factors attracting people to private work and those that repel them from it.

FANTASIES: TEN ARGUMENTS IN FAVOR OF PRIVATE PRACTICE

What is it that makes people opt for the private sector when there are perfectly good jobs out there within large organizations? When someone else is prepared to take all the risk and pay a reliable salary, why on earth would people look elsewhere?

No Big-Organization Hassles

> *If I obeyed every organizational rule, attended every committee meeting, and went through "proper channels" for everything, I would never see a client again! It's driving me crazy, and I just want out, into the clear, blue sky of private work, where no one tells you what to do.*

You might think money would be the number-one reason why people want to open their own businesses. It isn't. Frustrations with administrative inertia and incompetence are the most commonly cited motives. The issues include:

- Endless organizational meetings that decide nothing and seem to serve no useful purpose, but which one is not permitted to ignore

- Union rules that make staffing and job stability a matter of seniority rather than competence

- Zero-based budgeting, a system developed with the admirable goal of weeding out obsolete services, but with the primary results being days spent reediting the previous year's plea and a complete inability to plan beyond year-end

- Nonclinical administrators who have ultimate responsibility for programs despite never seeming to remember anything about them

- Regulations in which clinicians are compelled to join multidisciplinary unions that often have little desire to defend or even understand the interests of a smallish group of its higher-paid members

- Organization-wide accounting panics in which budget cuts or unexpected deficits mean that senior management staff hunt for any employee or program that can be cut to save money

- Productivity initiatives in which professionals are required to record the nature of their activities every fifteen minutes—a system with limited investigative utility, given that people typically complete their own record keeping (often simply making up the figures at the end of each reporting period)

- Being told to "embrace rather than fear change," despite knowing that many changes have more to do with new managers placing their stamps on their empires than any real improvement in service, and that many changes are made capriciously and without consultation

In the face of such circumstances, it can be hard to retain a sense that your work is valued and your job is secure. Planning for the future inevitably takes on a futile cast given that, at any moment, decisions from above can sweep away your work, your program, or your career. Should staff describe such an atmosphere as anything other than "exciting" or "dynamic," they are viewed as obstructionist or disloyal. No wonder so many professionals feel as if they are serving as faceless extras in a live stage production of Terry Gilliam's dystopian film *Brazil*, longing for the winged freedom that private practice might represent.

And just how valid is the fantasy? According to most private practitioners, 100 percent. Shifting to private practice means no more mandatory committee meetings, no one else responsible for the budget, no staff bumping, no union–management discord, and no helpless anxieties that the program will be cut through administrative error, organizational whim, or departmental reshuffling.

Getting Away from the Medical Model of Distress

> *The public system seems wedded to a medical approach that views human distress as a disorder, something like diabetes or the mumps, something that happens to people spontaneously and needs the miracles of chemistry to correct. I'm fed up.*

Many clinicians feel compelled by their organizations to participate in the propagation of an idea they see as a myth: that human distress is an illness needing to be treated, one that has nothing to teach us and provides no useful guidance or information about our lives. While this model may fit some disorders, it seems to have less relevance when the problem is mild-to-moderate depression, burnout, adjustment disorder, or general life dissatisfaction.

Participation in public service and large organizations affords clinicians the opportunity to question and shift the dominant model. In team meetings we can ask inconvenient questions, such as "But wouldn't depressed mood be a normal reaction for someone in this client's life situation, rather than evidence of a mysterious chemical imbalance?" But there are limits. Eventually we may want to abandon ship, erase the brick-wall indentations from our foreheads, and do something that seems more in line with both data and reality.

And…? Sure enough, private practice does enable us to throw off the burdens of organizational health care, and sometimes it's only then that we become aware of how heavy that weight was. It feels almost sinful to be able to practice our profession without arguing about it with our supervisors.

The freedom of private practice should not be overstated, however. Many clients are likely to be referred by physicians, employee assistance firms, or disability insurers. They will want to know diagnoses and may hope to guide the kind of treatment you provide. To receive reimbursement, clients may need to have you report to rehabilitation consultants, third-party payers, or other professionals, which may limit your freedom.

Increased Accessibility for Clients

I run a specialized service, but it's available to people only in my catchment area, only if they were previously hospitalized, only if the family physician refers them, and only if the consulting psychiatrist agrees. It doesn't much matter what the client wants, and if they live on the far side of Spruce Street, it doesn't matter what anyone thinks.

In many public or corporate organizations, access to mental health services has less to do with the individual's need than with various extraneous factors. The individual must live in the facility's catchment area, for example. If the person lives even one street over the border or has a different insurer, she must seek help through a different agency, even if that agency does not offer the services required.

In private practice, these concerns vanish. The practitioner is free to see anyone, diagnosed or not, insured or not, previously hospitalized or not, and from as far away as the client is willing to travel. Clients need not pass any diagnostic or professional hurdles, nor need they languish on a waiting list for months until they are seen.

It's not all roses in private practice, however. Practitioners impose their own admission criteria based on their interests and qualifications. As well, the issue of payment can be a major barrier (about which I will say more later). For the most part, these are challenges for the client seeking care, however, not for the clinician contemplating private practice. The organizational barriers that clinicians struggle against in institutional settings are, for the most part, removed.

You Get to See Whom You Want

No more managers foisting clients on me that I'm not interested in seeing, or problems that I'm not really competent to treat. If I'm in private practice, I'm in charge, and I get to decide on the population.

In private practice you can decide whom you will take, what problems you will treat, and for how long you will see people. You always have the option of turning down a referral, and no one else forces you to do anything.

This freedom is not absolute, however. The restrictions of management are replaced by the restrictions of the market and your ability to attract the people you hope to see.

Do you have a great love of trichotillomania? Terrific. Be sure you advertise this. But you'll starve if that's all you want to see. Even if you live in a major population center, you will never get close to having a majority of your referrals with any one concern, for the simple reason that providers refer mostly to the people they know, not the people who are the leading experts in obscure areas of practice.

Business is very different from professional school. In the academic setting, perhaps the primary consideration is *What interests me?* In the business world, the primary consideration has to be *What interests my customer?* Our passions are not irrelevant. They can indicate where we would most like to practice and perhaps what we will be best at. But they cannot blind us to what people actually want.

There's something fundamental about the shift from a professional orientation to a customer-centered perspective. If the clinic is about us, we will focus entirely on what we want and what works for us, rather than on what the client wants or has a right to expect. Imagining things from the client's (or referral source's) perspective can be a powerful way of enhancing the services we provide.

So yes, you ultimately decide what you will do. But there are limits that you may not perceive from the perspective of professional school or publicly funded health care.

More Money

> *In the public sector you start out doing quite well, but you top out early. Once you've been there ten years, you're making about as much as you ever will— unless you stop doing what you're good at and take up administration. I want to earn more by using my skills.*

No one goes into counseling or coaching because it seems like a ticket to riches; or if they do, they are deluded. Let's presume that no reader of this book has ever been so foolish. But money is undeniably a powerful reinforcer.

There is a cognitive trap out there, obvious to anyone who sits and thinks about it for a moment. Look at the hourly pay rates for any type of public service (or, for that matter, private companies, such as employee assistance firms). Then look at the fees charged by private practitioners with the same qualifications: it is often three to five times as much. Visions of country estates, yachts and butlers, limousines and moonlit Majorca nights dance through your head.

The two pay rates are not comparable, however. The hourly rate in most services is paid regardless of what you're doing: seeing clients, making notes, sitting in meeting rooms listening to your colleagues' vacation stories, perusing the referral list, scratching your nose. In private practice you get paid only for the hours you actually see clients, and perhaps for writing the odd report. Furthermore, at a regular paid position, you are given full salary for all statutory holidays and for several weeks of vacation each year. In private practice, every day you take off is a day you earn absolutely nothing. And from your earnings, you must subtract your entire overhead: lease, furniture, office supplies, licenses, assistants, and more miscellaneous items than you can imagine.

What do you actually take home? The leftovers. If you don't watch it, there won't be any of those. Every crumb will have been licked from the floor by your Internet supplier, your printing house, your telecom provider. And if they still aren't satisfied, they'll start going through your pockets, taking money you haven't actually earned. You can wind up paying more in overhead than you take in, subsidizing your clinic for the privilege of spending your life there.

So, is the goal of making more money a mistake? No, it's still possible to increase your income above that paid in regular salaried positions—in some cases markedly so. But to accomplish this, you'll have to do much more than come up with a pretty logo. It takes careful planning.

Supplement Your Salaried Income

> *I make a good salary, let's face it. But I do the math and realize I can add a lot to it without much more work. I just want a little extra income to let me do what I like.*

Aha, now these people are really thinking. One of the best business strategies for opening a private practice is to use it as an add-on to regular employment. There are lots of advantages to this:

- You don't give up the security of a regular paycheck. If the private practice doesn't take off, there's no real problem.

- You can often use your regular office for your private practice after hours. Any overhead charged will be a steal compared to what you would pay if you hung out an independent shingle.

- You can work your way up. Because you aren't diving headlong into practice, you can start slowly—even with just a single client—and gradually expand.

- You can start writing off professional expenses immediately, in many cases reducing the taxable portion of your first few clients to zero.

Money doesn't remember where it came from. But many professionals with a small private practice dedicate their private revenue to specific causes: "If I'm going to work late two evenings a week, I'm going to put all of that money aside to reward myself." The excess can be devoted to paying off your mortgage, funding travel to enjoyable conventions, making a down payment on a cottage, taking golf lessons, donating to an environmental charity—whatever you like.

Flexible Hours and Holidays

> *I'm fed up with having to work the same hours as everyone else just because the organization wills it. I want to spend time with my family, see a bit more of the world, and devote myself to things other than therapy. I want more than just two weeks of vacation.*

There's no question that private practice will allow you to decide when and how much you will work. Feel like an easier few days next week? Just schedule fewer clients or put off your paperwork for a while. Want to work four days rather than five? No one will object. Want to work Tuesday evenings, and start Wednesdays at one o'clock? Many of your clients will be delighted.

Of course, there are limits. Regular clients will expect to meet with you at the same time each week, so it's hard to shift your schedule on a whim. And if you sublet your office on the days you're not around, it can be difficult to change from week to week.

What about holidays? Rather than take off just two to four weeks a year, you can take as many holidays as you like. But you won't earn anything when you're out of the office. Taking a Wednesday off to go hiking is no longer a free day. If you usually see five clients at $150 each, it's a $750 hike. Is it worth that much to you? Unless you learn to accept these trade-offs, the opening day of your private practice will signal the end of your holidays—at least until you burn out and close your practice to recover.

So a requirement for private practitioners is to make a specific, concrete plan for how many holidays they *must* take and how many they *may* take, and to consciously let go of their fantasies about how much they could make if only they could be in the office all the time.

Work Fewer Hours

> *My work is my life, and I'm becoming more and more aware of how wrong that is for me. In therapy I'm all about balance, balance, balance, but I don't really have any balance in my own life. By the time I get home, I feel used up, and it takes me all weekend just to recover.*

A lot of therapists and coaches spend their days pointing out to clients that working seventy hours a week is seldom the path to fulfillment. Eventually the realization dawns that perhaps that haggard face in the mirror could use the same advice. Many agencies demand long hours of overtime, often unpaid, from their clinicians. It can be hard to saunter home when a suicidal teenager has just been admitted to the ward, a colleague begs you to cover for him during a leave, or a seriously ill person is deteriorating while on the waiting list. The desire to have more balance in your life, and particularly to work fewer hours, can be a major draw of private work.

The reality? Most clinicians report that private practice does allow them to work less than in a full-time regular position—if they choose to do so. The increased pay can allow for fewer hours, and there's no boss to dictate how many hours you should work. But much of your overhead (lease, equipment, phones, and more) will be the same regardless of how many clients you see. As well, no one will order you to go home or take a day off unless you have an unusually motherly assistant. The work limit will depend entirely on your own ability to set and maintain a boundary for yourself, in the face of the knowledge that if you were to see just one more client a week, that would be—let's see—the equivalent of a third of your mortgage.

When working for a big organization, we can salivate over the freedom of being our own boss. We fail to realize that for most clinicians, the superego, our sense of inadequacy, or the fear of bankruptcy can be a significantly more fearsome taskmaster than any program manager ever was.

No Commute!

> *Where I work now is an hour of highway driving from home. I feel like I'm wasting my life in a car and doing more damage to the environment than my job merits. I want to work closer to home.*

In 2003 the average American worker spent 48.6 minutes commuting each workday (U.S. Census Bureau, 2005). In Canada in 2005, the figure was 63 minutes (Turcotte, 2006). Assuming there are about 230 working days per year (including holidays and days off due to illness), this translates to between 23 and 30 eight-hour workdays spent in transit.

One rationale for many people who wish to open a private practice is the desire to work closer to home and spend less time in the car. Of the people I interviewed, none opted for a private practice farther from home than their previous job.

Unless you open an office in your home (a strategy that has its own drawbacks), you will still have a commute of some sort in a private practice. But opening a practice affords you the option of selecting a location reasonably close to home.

A Service Based on Your Own Vision

> *Ever since graduate school, I've had a dream of the kind of service I'd like to offer, but working at the agency has never given me enough freedom to do it. If I were in charge, I could finally create what I want.*

As we go through our training, we inevitably ask ourselves the childhood question, *What would I like to be when I grow up?*

At moments all things seem possible, but much of the time we are acutely aware that our dreams depend on the world rearranging itself to accommodate us.

We start out with our supervision requirements, our insecurities, our student loans. We set aside our fantasies to find somewhere, anywhere, that will take us in and give us a paycheck. The fit is never perfect. The agency specifically excludes our favorite population; the director favors an approach that we question; the team members are not to our liking. As time passes, we begin to fantasize about what we really wanted, why we really went into the field, and a new image based on experience starts to form: the ideal service, the fulfilling life.

For many of us, there will never be a perfect place for us in a puzzle of anyone else's making. We will have to create it ourselves.

Private practice may not be perfect either. We will have to worry about money. We may not be able to build the facility we really want. The demand may not be sufficient to sustain us. But it will be ours—however small, however modest. Within financial and professional limits, we can create what we want and sink or swim as a result. We can build a professional home for ourselves where no one can tell us what to do. And ultimately it is this that can make private practice so satisfying.

So why not try it? Well...

FEARS: TEN ARGUMENTS AGAINST PRIVATE PRACTICE

Even some of the fantasies have their limitations. But what often holds people back from private practice is fear. As in the rest of life, some of our fears are valid, based on a clear-eyed assessment of reality. Some are invalid projections of our own insecurities or are founded on misinformation. Let's look at the most common drawbacks as experienced by those contemplating the leap.

You'll Never Get Clients

So, let's say I get a place, get all set up, and open my doors. What if no one comes? I'll go broke.

If you sat down right now and totaled your expenses—your mortgage or rent, your car payments and maintenance, your food, your lifestyle—it would probably amount to a fair bit of money. If you're contemplating a part-time private practice, perhaps you won't depend on it for all of those needs. But if you want a full-time practice, your clients will have to pay for every stick of furniture, every meal at every restaurant, every grain of rice, every ounce of gas—and all of that will come out of the revenue left over once your private-practice expenses are paid.

If you start your full-time practice from nothing, it's unlikely that your schedule will fill during the first week—or month. And if you sit at your desk waiting, the phone is unlikely to ring. But if you follow fairly standard and understandable procedures for enhancing referral flow, you will probably find that clients begin to trickle in. As they spread the word to their friends and back to the referral source, more will come. Most people find that referrals are slow at first, but eventually their practices become well established. If referrals dry up, a few basic moves will often nudge open the faucet again.

You're No Good at Networking or Marketing

I've always felt disdain for real estate agents and insurance salesmen, smiling broadly and handing over their cards at parties. I can't do that. I'd want to take a bath afterward. And I'll never be able to spout off about how great I am and why people should come see me.

Few counselors or psychotherapists are natural entrepreneurs. Despite spending their lives talking to people, most are relatively shy individuals, not predisposed to self-promotion. Their training usually offers them little guidance about becoming established, and they often snobbishly imagine that they are above all that sales work anyway. So the task is doubly difficult: not only do they need to learn skills that were not on their original curriculum, they have to get past their disdain for the whole concept of marketing.

You will have to acknowledge that your practice is a business. As in any business, you are selling things. Imagine tending a market stall and hiding your wares under the table. Perhaps your pottery is the most beautiful, your scarves are the brightest and softest, your apples the most flavorful—irrelevant; the stall next door will sell far more than you ever do. You would snort at the foolishness of any vendor who behaved this way, but you might regard such actions as the height of professionalism for any counselor. You're going to have to get over that view.

Most people at my workshops report experiencing anxiety about self-promotion but were able to overcome it enough to do at least a little of it. This seemed to be enough. No one proclaimed their stunning skill at networking, but most reported that their practices filled anyway. When the average level of promotional skill in the field is as low as it is, there is a huge opportunity available to anyone willing to make an effort.

Uncertainty About Income from Month to Month

My bills are steady. The bank expects the same mortgage payment every month. I eat about the same, use the same phone, and heat my place to the same temperature. So I'd like some reliability in my paycheck, and I worry that in private practice, I won't get it.

People worry that when they start out, their referrals will come in haltingly: one month flood, the next month drought. The reality is that private practices work like this even after they've been established for years. You seem to be the flavor of the month, getting more referrals than you can comfortably handle. Then, without warning, the phone stops ringing.

Every private practitioner I've spoken to reports this phenomenon, and few of us have anything other than superstitious ideas about why it happens: "Maybe it's my lucky socks." One year you think you've figured out that referrals dry up once the nice weather starts; the next year you're inundated come spring.

After a few of these waves, you will begin hoarding clients the way a squirrel hoards nuts. When the flood comes, you'll try to handle everyone, inflating your therapy hours beyond the burnout point, fearful that soon the river will run dry. When the fax machine cools off, you'll spend inordinate amounts of time brainstorming new marketing techniques, drafting letters to your referral sources announcing almost anything to remind them that you exist: "Mountainview Clinic proudly reports that we have purchased a new water cooler for the benefit of our clients." Then before you mail any of them out, the phone starts ringing again.

The voice of experience will not tell you why this happens, just that it does. The mission is to ride the waves and not panic when you feel the tide of popularity receding.

You Hate All the Clerical and Business Demands

I want to be a clinician, not a business owner.
I don't know enough about accounting or office
management, and I don't want to learn.

When you work for a large organization, there are people who can help you organize your life. Receptionists book your clients, the records department handles your files, the accounting department issues your pay, plant services deals with the heating and air conditioning, and human resources figures out your benefits.

In private practice you're in charge of every department. You choose the size of cups for the water cooler, you set the room temperature, you shop for the chairs, you wire up the printer—unless and until you hire other people to perform at least some of these functions.

This is a genuine drawback of private practice, one that many people forget when contemplating their departure from a larger organization. Administrative demands can be endless and unrelenting. If you aren't careful, you can wind up spending half your time dealing with clerical minutiae and not getting paid for doing so. Private work will involve getting past your reluctance, learning basic business practices, and developing systems for tasks as basic as making a bank deposit. Failure to pay attention to this side of the work probably accounts for more private-practice failures than anything else.

You Don't Know Enough to Practice Independently

I'm okay when I'm working as part of a group, but I rely on the chance to consult with colleagues. In a private practice I'd be all on my own, and I just don't feel confident that I'd know all that I needed to know.

Good for you for thinking this. You're right. You don't know enough to work independently—and you never will. The dangerous practitioners are the ones who think they understand it all. They are like demented sailors; they put their practice on a set course and then sit blindfolded at the tiller in utmost confidence until they or their clients hit the rocks.

I am often troubled at the thought of newly minted clinicians, fresh out of graduate school, who set up an independent practice right away. They start working based on textbook knowledge and highly structured training experiences and have no real idea what they don't know. They have no professional network of colleagues to depend on and consult with, and they often cover their anxieties with secrecy and hope for the best.

Experience in a larger organization or a group practice is invaluable prior to setting out in your own private practice. You can build a network on which you will rely for advice and referrals when you leave. Meanwhile, you consult with them informally and in team meetings or rounds, learning not only how to handle difficult client features but also how to approach a problem and resolve it. This is invaluable and perhaps indispensable.

People never reach the point where they are ready for completely independent work, and they are kidding themselves if they think otherwise. Consequently, one of the challenges of setting up a practice is to figure out how to consult with colleagues when they aren't sitting down the hall. Many private practitioners form consultation groups that meet regularly, discuss professional issues or difficult cases, and provide the opportunity for input from divergent perspectives. Between meetings, members can call or e-mail each other for more immediate advice as needed.

One thing you cannot do is master everyone else's profession or specialty in addition to your own. One profession is more than enough to occupy anyone's brain, and if you study from now until the end of time, you'll never really learn all there is to know. So there's no point in adding more fields to a plate that is already overflowing with undigested knowledge. Instead, develop a network of professionals you can consult with, either formally or informally.

Where will you get them? Most private practitioners start out in some kind of larger organization and, in the course of their work, develop collegial relationships with a variety of other people. If you call up your old buddies, they are likely to feel flattered rather than exploited. Don't waste their time, don't overstay your welcome on the phone, and don't ask them about trivia you could easily look up. But do feel free to contact people and ask them questions. Ever since Delphi, most of us have longed to be the oracle. When an old friend puts us in that position, we tend to take it as a compliment.

Dealing with Fees Will Be a Huge Hassle

> *I'm used to seeing people and providing service, not demanding to be paid. I'll hate asking for money from clients who are poorer than I am, and I'll feel a constant pressure to make sure I give them their money's worth every session.*

When you work in a setting where other people deal with billing and budgets, you have the luxury of focusing all of your efforts on delivering services. You are like a therapeutic Santa Claus, giving and asking nothing in return—at least not directly. This can feel virtuous and has the added benefit of alleviating anxiety about whether you are offering full value. If a session with a client seems to tread water without making much progress, well, not much is lost for the client other than an hour out of her day.

In private practice you will ask for payment each session. Part of your brain will always be weighing the exchange: *Did I give enough to merit the amount I am charging?* The "good" you provide usually can't be measured. Even if your psychometrics show an improvement, perhaps the client would have gotten better anyway with the passage of time.

Consequence? Anxiety about asking for money. Perhaps you will be embarrassed to ask for so much. Perhaps you will feel tempted to reduce the rate for an unproductive session. Or maybe the client will look at you and remark that you aren't worth your pay.

How do you resolve these anxieties in advance of opening your private practice? You don't. You accept the anxiety as part of the price of the work, at least in the first days and weeks. It doesn't last forever. There's a reason why exposure therapy is a staple of anxiety treatment: it works. Do something you fear often enough, and you get used to it. Within a surprisingly short time, discussions about finances will roll off your tongue without embarrassment: "Would you like to deal with payment this session or next?" "Simon, our bill for last month hasn't been paid just yet; can you let me know when you will get to it?"

You'll Be Helpless in the Face of Insurers or Funders

I'll be one of a hundred small-practice providers, so why would a big insurer pay attention to any demands I make? There's no union to fall back on. They'll set the rates, they'll say what I do, and I'll just have to go along.

A lot of jobs in large organizations are unionized, which protects the workers from most kinds of unfair treatment. As well, the union theoretically takes on the responsibility of advocating for clinicians in terms of pay and working conditions. But there is also a frustration about unions, one that contributes to the attraction of private work for many clinicians. Merit is almost irrelevant. Pay scales, job security, and advancement opportunities are based almost entirely on seniority.

It's true that in private practice, there are no babysitters or pinch hitters to go to bat for you. But there is a meritocracy. Seniority counts for very little. Merit may be dispensed based more on practice management (the ability to promote, regular interactions with referral sources, prompt billing) than on therapeutic outcomes, but at least this places more control in your own hands.

Private practice doesn't mean you never have to deal with large organizations, however. Many referrals may come from insurers or large corporations, which often have strict policies about the rates they pay. You may be good at what you do, but this will not change the rate.

If you are dissatisfied, you can decline to offer your services under the terms specified. This may sound unrealistic given the need to make money, but in fact almost every provider does this with at least some potential referral sources. You can't turn everyone down, of course, and some people build their practices around one or two primary referral sources that would be difficult to do without. But the freedom to decline work is one of the undeniable pleasures of a successful private practice. The goal of producing enough business that you can decline some referrals is yet one more reason to conduct effective practice planning and management.

No Retirement Plan or Benefits

I basically keep working at the hospital for the benefits. I have kids, the kids have braces, and I have a health condition. Giving up a salaried job means giving up my safety net.

Sick days, short-term disability, long-term disability, pension plan, health insurance, dental plan, massage therapist coverage, counseling visits, family days, maternity leave, bereavement leave, life insurance—regular employment entails far more than a salary.

Full-time private practice involves giving up all of these benefits, at least as an automatic add-on to the job. The option of maintaining a benefits package is one of the main reasons people give for keeping a part-time salaried position rather than shifting altogether to private work.

The financial constraints that some people experience when starting a practice can encourage them to economize by going without benefits. They simply don't have the extra money, and eliminating that budget line enables them to maintain something closer to their old salary. But many professional organizations have arranged for benefits packages for private practitioners, and it can be a good idea to purchase these.

As well, it is even more important in private practice than in salaried full-time employment to start contributing to your own retirement savings plan as soon as possible and to make this a top spending priority. The best strategy is the automatic monthly contribution, in which a set amount is shifted from your bank account to your retirement plan before you ever see it, mimicking the way retirement savings happen in most salaried positions.

You'll Burn Out and Won't Have a Safety Net

> *If I get overwhelmed or stressed out at work, I can scale back a bit, drop a few committees, and recover. In private practice I won't have the luxury of slowing down, and the demand to perform will push me to the breaking point; then there'll be nothing to catch me.*

This is a reality held in utmost secrecy by many individuals in health care. Their own functioning fluctuates from month to month or season to season. Sometimes they feel full of optimism and energy, ready to take on and execute new projects. Sometimes they get overwhelmed, their energy declines, and it becomes more difficult to handle all of their commitments. Salaried positions often shield people from this problem. If you become overwhelmed, you can slough off some commitments, ride out the low, and then get more ambitious once your energy returns.

In private practice this is more difficult. If you reduce your client load, you reduce your income—and a disappointed loan officer can be just as daunting as a frustrated boss. If you maintain your client load but cut back on administrative work, you will feel your service sinking gently but relentlessly into disorganization and dysfunction.

Does this mean that people prone to somewhat variable efficiency should avoid private practice altogether? No. You can build buffers into your practice that allow for some breathing space. One of the most essential is to budget your life for less than your average income. If your service has to be full to the brim to pay the bills, then you cannot cut back. You will be a slave to the practice rather than its master.

Like everyone else, we should pay attention to occasional declines in our energy or capacity and use them as welcome cues to take care of ourselves: ramp up our exercise, refocus on the sustaining elements of our lives, determine where we have gone astray. We should create a life that acknowledges the reality that we are not machines and that we will not hum away contentedly at the same rate until we retire. Private practice gives us control over our demands, but only if we build the control into it.

You Won't Have a Sense of Meaning in Your Work

> *It won't be about the work anymore; it'll be about the money. I'll have to take anything at all just to ensure that I earn enough, and the first thought on my mind when someone talks to me will be* What can I make from this?

There is freedom in working for a big organization; freedom that often is not recognized until it is taken away. It is the freedom to focus on your core role without having to worry about money. In your spare time you might fret about your bills or wonder about opportunities for advancement. But while you are at work, your primary responsibility is to do your job, which is unlikely to have anything to do with collecting money for the organization.

By contrast, in private practice your attention is always split between providing services and ensuring the financial viability of the business. At times you may find that you need to accept business you would prefer not to have. Over time you run the risk of sliding down the slippery slope, attending more to financial considerations and less to the reasons you went into private work in the first place.

This problem illustrates yet again an important principle of private practice: all of the boundaries depend on you. No one will tell you to go home, take a vacation, see fewer clients, pay more attention to your billing practices, or prioritize your work. Although this affords you much more control, it also imposes a need for vigilance to ensure that your work conforms at least partially to your vision while enabling you to remain solvent.

In a sense, private practice is vocational adulthood. In my own career, I had the option of pursuing an academic tenure-track life or leaving the university gates. Staying at the university felt too much like never leaving home, sacrificing my freedom for the comforts of having someone else do my laundry and cook for me. This was in large part what led me to work outside the academic setting. I didn't realize it at the time, but private practice was yet another step away from the cradle, a frightening but ultimately fulfilling one.

The balance between the attractions and repulsions of private practice differ for everyone based on temperament, ambitions, talents, and life circumstances. By its nature, private practice is not a unified beast, a career slot into which you may or may not fit. It is variable, subject to tailoring, and adaptable to the needs of the individual. Beyond the decision of whether or not to pursue private work is the more complicated question of how to structure it to suit your own preferences and vision. Thus, there are as many types of private practice as there are practitioners.

Nevertheless, there are commonalities: boundaries that define the field and guidelines that can help maximize success. In the chapters to come, we will discuss them with the goal of tilting the balance, not only from repulsion to attraction but also from anxiety to fulfillment.

CHAPTER 2

Who/Where: Names and Location

Yes or no? This is the fence that prospective private practitioners sit on, sometimes for years. Once the balance has tilted toward yes, the issues become more complicated. In this chapter we consider the questions of whom to see and where to see them.

WHO: DECIDING ON THE NATURE OF YOUR PRACTICE

Perhaps you already know what you want to do with your practice: whom you want to see, how you want to structure it. But let's nail it down a bit.

Age Groups

Traditionally therapists talk about four age groups: children, adolescents, adults, and seniors. Let's consider them in descending age order with regard to private practice.

SENIORS

Working with seniors involves helping them deal with specific issues, including adjustment to retirement, chronic-illness concerns, the concept of developmental stage (often emphasizing generativity), end-of-life issues, grief and loss concerns, cognitive ability questions, and more. Few practitioners exclude this population from their private practices. If you plan to see seniors, however, it is useful to be aware of their special issues with regard to the difficulties you treat. Depression, for example, may manifest differently or have different causes in seniors. You will also want to be particularly concerned with access issues for people with mobility problems. If you specialize in helping seniors, you may find you have a niche almost to yourself, as this is a rarity in counseling practice.

ADULTS

The largest population of consumers for private practice, adults also attract the most practitioners—in some regions, more than the numbers warrant. If you work mainly with adults, you may need to spend more time defining and marketing your specialties than professionals who work primarily with one of the other age groups.

ADOLESCENTS

Despite occupying a narrow age band, adolescents are a surprisingly large population among therapy referrals. They often bring particular psychological challenges: emotional lability, self-centered myopia, unwarranted self-confidence combined with poor decision-making skills, vulnerability to conformity pressure from peers, nascent autonomy producing an oppositional stance to external guidance, initial forays into the worlds of romance and sex, and so on.

Systemically there are challenges as well: adolescents may seek treatment primarily because their parents see a problem that they themselves dismiss; parents often expect the therapist to toe the parental line or to provide progress updates; school authorities and others often stir the pot; the client seldom pays for the service and so has limited investment in its success; and so forth.

Consequently, many practitioners avoid adolescent clients, creating a service vacuum that is potentially advantageous for those willing (and hopefully eager) to see teens. Expertise in developing an effective alliance with younger clients is particularly valuable, and a firm grasp of regional legislation about confidentiality and reporting are essential.

CHILDREN

Children are usually thought to represent a specialty that's separate from the rest of clinical practice. A population underserved by private practitioners in many regions, children can provide an excellent focus for a successful clinic. Those wishing to see children will have to keep the population in mind when choosing and furnishing clinic space. Offices may need to be somewhat bigger, for example, to accommodate children and parents and to provide play space. Soundproofing may also be a bigger issue than for therapists who see only adults.

Populations Seen

The opportunity to target specific client groups is one of the prime attractions of private practice, without which many clinicians would choose to continue working for larger organizations. Your choices may influence where you locate your office or the type of office you seek. If your specialty is spinal cord injury, you will want to be particularly certain that your space is wheelchair friendly. If you speak Tagalog and want to serve the Filipino community, it will be important to know whether there is a concentration of Filipinos in one part of the city. If you want to conduct family therapy, you will need larger consulting rooms.

Take some time to write down all of the types of work you imagine yourself doing and for which you have training. Consider characteristics of both the client and the type of service you would like to offer. Here are some suggestions (most are general categories; be more specific if you can):

Specific diagnostic categories	End-of-life issues
Addictions	Custody and access
Issues related to sexuality or orientation	Women's or men's issues
	Forensic work
Linguistic or ethnic origin groups	Vocational counseling
	Workplace mental health issues
Sensory or motor disabilities	Life, executive, or lifestyle coaching
Relationship, parenting, or family counseling	
	Faith-based counseling
Neuropsychology	Sports psychology
Coping with health problems	Specific therapy/counseling models
Reproductive issues	
Educational assessment/counseling	

Note that your fantasy population may entail a combination of categories: life coaching for hearing-impaired women, cognitive therapy for depressed gay athletes. Every specifier shrinks the population, making clients more difficult to find and increasing the importance of both marketing and having a list of specialties rather than just one.

When you have your list, consult an Internet-based referral service for your profession. Pick a reasonably random subset of twenty to thirty providers (perhaps last names from A to C) and tabulate how many see something close to each of your specialties. For particularly specific concerns (services offered in Swedish, for example), search the entire list for other providers. Consider what you know about the demand for each service. If there appears to be no competition, this may mean that you will have the turf all to yourself, or it may mean that there is no market. If there are many providers offering the same service, you may need to find some way to distinguish yourself from the pack.

Whatever you decide, recognize that in your previous position, you may have developed a considerable thirst for work with a specific population. This can cause you to overestimate your interest, just as overwork causes many people to imagine they would be happy fishing every day. If you suffer from Oscar Wilde's tragedy of getting what you wish for, you may discover that a balance between several interests would be preferable to a career of just one flavor. Having a range of activities and services you can offer will enhance both your marketability and your endurance.

Exclusionary Factors

You have bright spots of expertise and interest within the galaxy of opportunity, but you also have black holes of incompetence and aversion. It is worthwhile to identify the areas in which you do not intend to practice so you can screen out certain referrals before wasting anyone's time or money.

A professional at a recent workshop stated he had happily treated child abusers until he himself had children, at which point he became completely ineffective with this population. Another provider said she had to cut back sharply on her work with distressed couples when her own marriage encountered difficulty. A gay psychologist felt unable to handle too many HIV cases due to his own past losses.

Regardless of your life situation, there are probably areas where you are ineffective. Certain disorders may seem opaque to you; you find it difficult to gain any real understanding of them. Without an instinctive sense of a difficulty, it is hard to practice therapy effectively. Anorexia is one such problem for many male providers, violently abusive men an example for many more. Some people develop a real "feel" for autism, whereas others cannot relate to it at all.

Still, more areas are simply outside the scope of your training. Substance abuse may be prevalent, but perhaps you know too little about it to be useful to people in its grip. Couples counseling is a specialty all its own, and if you know too little, you will simply fall into the trap of deciding which person is more in the right.

You may be reluctant to identify exclusionary factors for your practice, because in doing so, you are effectively acknowledging your own incompetence, which is rarely a loved task. As well, you cut yourself off from a potential source of income, while wondering whether what remains will be enough to sustain you. Nevertheless, any shopkeeper must come to terms with what her store does not stock and won't attempt to sell. Consider taking some time to make a list of the populations and issues you already know you wouldn't want to see, or with whom you know you would not work effectively.

Group or Individual Therapy?

Most private practitioners see people individually, but many wish to offer group interventions for a variety of reasons. They may have developed expertise in group work and don't want to let their skills languish. Offering both group and individual therapy can be a way to diversify and stay fresh. Group therapy can be cheaper for clients, thus reducing a barrier to services. Groups can be as or more effective than individual therapy for some problems (clients with panic disorder, for example, often gain considerable inspiration from watching others' improvements). Group therapy can enable therapeutic tasks to take place during the therapy session (clients with social phobia can practice relating with others, clients with germ phobias can shake hands, and everyone can address intimacy and privacy issues).

Groups can pose difficulties, however. They require a larger space than many clinicians have available. It can be difficult to recruit enough people all at once. Billing can be an issue, because if enough clients drop out of your group, you will wind up earning less than you would if you were seeing people individually.

One way to make groups more workable is to shift from a closed-ended to an open-ended group model. An open-ended group still necessitates having enough clients at the outset, but you can add people later and replace your graduates. You won't be stuck seeing the three people left in your group while juggling the eight waiting in line for the next program. Most structured group protocols can be adapted fairly easily to the open-group format. As well, open groups give longer-term group members the opportunity to hear the same concepts a second time and perhaps to offer confidence-building guidance to the newbies.

If you think you would like to run groups, it is best to consider this carefully before you rent space. It will be difficult to add a group room to your facility later on.

Naming Your Practice

Eventually you need to name your practice. Some people get by with their own names: Anne Singh, registered psychologist. But perhaps you would like something a bit more descriptive, or perhaps you anticipate inviting colleagues to join you as the service ramps up. Jason Chen will not want to be known as Anne Singh Incorporated, and you'll need something to put on the letterhead and the voice-mail message. Here are some guidelines.

Don't name it after your street or neighborhood. What if you move or open a second office? The Mississauga Clinic will be confusing and out of place in Scarborough, and clients may skip over your service in a directory, assuming you are located where the name implies.

Don't name it after you and your partner. Chen and Singh Psychological Services may sound great, but what happens when Singh goes off on her own? Either you stick with what is now a misleading name, or you tear up all the cards and letterhead and start again.

Make it easy to spell. Quattrociacchi Counseling may look good to you, but people will curse the spelling for as long as you are in business, and they will never find your website. If your own name is difficult to spell, this is a good reason to find an alternative for your business name.

Make it memorable. Eventually you want your popularity to spread by word of mouth, but this won't happen if no one can remember your name. It should not be so generic that it's forgettable (Psychology Services, Inc.) or so esoteric that it's confusing (The Center for Metatheoretical Modeling).

Make it short. The Rothstein Center for Cognitive Behavioral Management of Psychological Difficulty may sound great, but no one will use the full name. If the name is longer than three words, it should make a memorable acronym. RCCBMPD doesn't cut it.

Don't name it after a psychological difficulty. Trichotillomania R Us may accurately reflect your core interest, but what if you want to see people with other issues? Does the Seattle Anxiety Clinic treat depression? It may, but it doesn't sound like it, so people with depression may look elsewhere.

The website name should be intuitive. You don't want people to have to do a Web search every time they go to your site. Create a name that easily translates to a Web address, make sure the domain is available for purchase, and buy it as soon as possible. In my case, Changeways Clinic became www.changeways.com.

Some jurisdictions or regulatory agencies impose restrictions on what you can call your service. You may be compelled by your professional association to use your own name or your partners' names. This seems like a needless overregulation of the profession, providing limited utility for the protection of the public. But if you have to, you have to.

Assessment Practice or Therapy Practice?

Some people prefer the variety, diagnostic challenge, and smaller emotional involvement of an assessment-only practice. People get referred, they come in, you see them for a few hours, you sit back with a cup of tea and write a report for someone, and it's on to the next file. You have less involvement in people's lives or traumas, so you run less risk of taking their problems home with you. Solving the problem is explicitly not part of the job description, so you don't have to worry too much about becoming overinvested in outcomes. Someone else takes ultimate responsibility for the client, so there are few emergencies. Planning for vacations is easier because you are not interrupting a long-term therapy sequence.

The downside? You never see the end of the story, and you may feel that you are simply identifying the problem rather than helping to solve it. You don't see anyone for long, so you need a constant stream of new referrals. You can begin seeing your work as an assembly line where you simply churn out report after report. You may wonder whether your recommendations are ever followed.

The other option is to offer assessment and treatment, in which you evaluate the client's difficulty, then create and carry out a plan of care. This enables you to follow up on your own findings. The reporting requirements are often less onerous, because you communicate with other caregivers only on an as-needed basis, and usually they don't expect a multipage report. You get the satisfaction of a deeper connection with your clients. You see the outcomes of your own recommendations (for good or ill). And you keep clients for a somewhat longer time, meaning your referral rate need not be as brisk.

Some practitioners prefer a combination of short-term assessments and longer-term therapy cases. If you go this route, you don't have to decide on your ideal mix before opening your practice. But you should have some idea of your preferences before drawing up your pamphlets, practice announcements, and website.

Short-Term or Long-Term Therapy?

Would you prefer to conduct longer-term interventions or short-term therapy? In part, of course, the answer will depend on the populations you see. Some issues require more time than others, and different clients with the same condition may wish to approach their problems at a different pace. Some therapists prefer to focus intently on a small number of presenting problems. Others prefer to work on not only the problem at hand but also the surrounding context and background in which the client lives—a slower approach with a broader focus.

Shorter-term therapy has the advantage of a sharp focus on outcomes. It operates within your clients' financial constraints or that of their insurance coverage, and it suits the stated goals of many clients who enter therapy. It avoids the issue of therapy dependence.

Longer-term therapy enables a clinician to tolerate a lower referral rate. It can provide clients with time to reveal their most difficult experiences and consider fully the therapist's response to them. It allows for clients to engage in extended practice of new skills between sessions and to layer new skills atop one another (for example, a socially phobic client might progress from asking a question in class to presenting a seminar). But longer-term therapy also runs the risk of becoming a replacement for intimacy in the client's (and the therapist's) life. Making suffering tolerable through regular applications of support can reduce the motivation for change rather than facilitate change. Without targeted outcomes, therapy can go on endlessly, perseverating due to the unspoken and irrational belief that the cessation of all problems and distressing emotions will serve as the signal of therapy's completion.

WHERE: FINDING OFFICE SPACE

Some of the issues involved in defining the type of practice you want can be amorphous, theoretical, or contentious. The considerations involved in locating and choosing office space are typically more down to earth.

The Neighborhood

If you live in a community of any size, your office will be convenient to at least some clients, no matter where you are. This frees you up to base your decision in large part on your own preferences.

One issue is your commute. No one will have to go from home to your office as often as you do, so it is legitimate to base your decision partly on your own convenience. Perhaps you could open an office within walking distance of your home, neatly reducing your commute, shrinking your ecological footprint, and integrating exercise into your life all at the same time.

Another question is where your clients are located. If you want to serve the gay community, perhaps an office near the local gay village would enhance your practice. If you speak another language, consider a neighborhood where people who speak that language tend to live. If you have a large practice with the deaf, perhaps you could open your office beside a school or resource center for the deaf population. A practice focusing on a particular medical issue may benefit from a location near a hospital specializing in that disorder or field of practice.

You will also want your clinic to be accessible to the largest possible population. If you are located in the middle of a populated area, people can come from all directions to see you, and few will have to travel very far.

Take a look at zoning regulations. Some space is zoned for offices, some for light industry, some for heavy industry. In many communities, office-space zoning is further subdivided into different types.

39

Counseling or psychology clinics may be classified as health facilities, and they sometimes come with their own requirements (including the availability of parking). So don't waste your time drooling over that lovely loft space down in the warehouse section of town, at least until you have checked your city's zoning laws and found out whether you would be permitted to open your clinic there.

Look at transit access. Some clients will take transit, so it is ideal if you are located along a major route or beside a transportation hub, such as a subway station. The view may be better two blocks west, but the closer you are to the train or bus stop, the more people will think of your office as an easy place to get to.

Many clients will probably drive, so it is a good idea to be close to major roads that are not jammed with traffic. When they arrive at your clinic, clients will need a place to park. It is ideal if your building has a well-lit and inexpensive parking lot attached. If not, scout around to find other nearby lots, and note their rates. Being able to tell clients where they can find the best parking (and ensuring that your assistants can do so as well) can help generate a positive impression of your service.

What About a Home Office?

One way to lower your overhead is to work out of your own home, a strategy offering both advantages and disadvantages. First, the advantages:

- No office rental costs.

- No long-term lease locking you into the same space for years at a time.

- You have reasonable control over most aspects of the environment.

- You can possibly deduct part of your mortgage interest from your taxes.

- No commuting.
- You can simply go to the kitchen for lunch rather than hit a restaurant.
- Easy access to all of your records when you want to write up a report on the weekend.
- Potentially, a warm and cozy environment.

So far, a home office sounds pretty appealing. But there are significant disadvantages as well.

- Giving up a significant part of your home to your business.
- A lack of separation between home life and work life.
- Inadequate soundproofing.
- The need for a separate entrance to your office.
- Difficult clients know where you live.
- Clients can (and will) drive past while you are cutting the lawn in your sweatpants or drinking beer on your veranda.
- You must rely on your family members to maintain the professionalism of your office.

Perhaps the most significant disadvantages are the low-probability ones. What if a hostile client knows the identity of your family members? What if clients in distress pop by in the middle of the night? What if your children accidentally reveal the identity of one of your clients to someone? Even though these may be infrequent or unlikely events, they may outweigh the advantages of operating a home office.

The issue is moot for many practitioners in any case. Most communities have relatively strict zoning that does not permit health-service-related businesses in residential areas. You will need a business license to operate legally, and if you contravene zoning regulations, you are unlikely to be issued one. You will probably have a home office anyway: a place to write reports, read the research, and store old files. But if, rather than reserve it as a base for your paperwork, you have clients come to that office on a regular basis, the drawbacks more than outweigh the benefits in most cases.

Serviced Office Space

An alternative to leasing your own office is to sublet office space from a *turnkey office*. This is a large suite of offices operated by a single company, which then rents individual offices or office days out to various firms. Usually the owner provides a receptionist, waiting room, water cooler, fax machine, telephone service, mail service, and shipping and delivery desk. Your own clinic number rings through to the front desk, where the receptionist notes the number being called and answers with the name of your company: "Good morning, Adel Consulting Services…"

One option is to rent an office for your exclusive use. The space may come furnished or unfurnished and enables you to store all of your materials and files there, just as you would in a complete suite you leased yourself. The other option is to rent an office for a limited number of days per week.

Advantages of this kind of space over traditional leased suites include:

- You can start small and gradually add office days as your business grows. If you add other providers, you can often take a second office in the same space, whereas a traditional office suite is difficult to expand.

- The shorter lease requirement—sometimes just a few months, compared to three or more years with a regular office suite—makes it much easier to move or close down.

- You get reception services without having to hire your own receptionist.

- You get a waiting room and reception area shared with other tenants, thus avoiding the expense of renting waiting-room space that is usually empty in a therapist's clinic.

- The waiting room is typically a distance from your office, reducing concerns about your next client hearing the voice of the previous one.

- Your telephone is answered throughout office hours every day.

- Office maintenance is entirely managed by the rental company, taking this off your own responsibility list.

- You can rent space in several neighborhoods, thus creating a multiple-location service without renting whole suites in each region.

- Many suites have a bookable boardroom space you can use for larger meetings or even group therapy.

Disadvantages of these offices include:

- If you rent by the day, you may have to remove all of your files and supplies at each day's end.

- You may need a more extensive home office to make up for the lack of storage in the rental space.

- Decisions about furniture, waiting-room layout, and reception staffing are not your own to make.

- Your neighbors in the facility may influence your image.

- Serviced offices look less expensive and more temporary than if you have your own clinic, possibly making your service seem less well established and less prestigious.

On the whole, turnkey office space can be an excellent solution for professionals wanting to operate a part-time practice, those who would like to have several locations, and practitioners wanting an easy escape from private practice if it's not for them. If a turnkey office looks like an option for you, here are some recommendations:

- Check the identity of the other renters. Will they reflect badly on your own service?

- Ensure that the receptionist is familiar with the confidentiality requirements of counseling practices (for example, not loudly repeating a caller's name in earshot of people in the waiting room).

- Check on the quality of upkeep and services by asking other renters whether they are satisfied.

- Call one of the companies renting space there to get a feel for the receptionist's professionalism.

- Turnkey space will always seem much more expensive than leased space if you compare the square footage of the office. Remember that in a leased suite you would be paying for a waiting room, phone lines, receptionist, fax machine, water service, and so on. Include these costs in your comparison.

Qualities of the Building

Let's assume you have opted to lease your own space. Most buildings will post the name and number of the leasing agent if they have space available. Call and make an appointment. But what do you want to know? (An "Office Space Viewing Sheet" is available at the websites noted in the introduction.)

You want the building to be nice but not opulent. You're not an investment banker. Your goal is comfort, not awe. Clients want to sense that the clinic is not all about the money. Shabbiness is not the goal either; you want to communicate simplicity and calm, not slovenly inattention.

Is the building in a noisy area? Is the traffic heavy? Is it under a flight path or near a rail yard? Is it on a major emergency services route, where there will be constant sirens? Is the parking area open air, and will you hear car alarms every time they go off? What are the windows like: single- or double-glazed? Remember that in a noisy building, the agent may have arranged for you to view it at a quiet time of day.

Ask to look at the washrooms. Are they clean and well maintained? Given that a third to half of client visits will include a trip to the washroom, will the facilities reflect well on your clinic? Is there a keyed entry, and do the facilities appear to be reasonably safe?

Is the building wheelchair accessible? Ask the agent, but verify this yourself (or enlist the help of a disabled friend). What about the washrooms? Are there wheelchair-accessible washrooms on every floor or just one on a distant floor?

What are the building's hours? Most office buildings are not left open twenty-four hours a day. This is a good thing. You don't want people to come off the street on a Sunday afternoon and have all day to burgle the building. But if you work evenings or Saturdays, can your clients get in? Find out when the doors are locked, and verify that this is done reliably at the same time each weekday. You don't want your 5:30 p.m. client to encounter an unexpectedly locked door. Check on the parking-garage hours too. If the garage closes at 6:00 p.m. and you routinely book 5:30 p.m. appointments for the after-work crowd, you will have to warn those clients to park elsewhere.

Look at the building's entry system. How do people get in when the doors are locked? You may have a main door key or magnetic card for entry. Can you get additional copies of them, if needed, for your colleagues, your assistant, and perhaps the people to whom you sublet space? How would clients get in after hours? Most office buildings have an exterior buzzer system similar to apartment buildings. Some of these activate the elevator to allow the client to go only to your floor. If clients need to use a wheelchair-accessible washroom on another floor, how will they do that?

Look at the building directory and suite signage. Is the lobby directory neat and well maintained? How quickly would your information be entered on it? Does your lease cover this cost, or will you have to pay for it yourself? Are there additional directories in the elevators or on parking levels? How do they look? What about signage at the suite door? How many lines of text can you have? Is this included in the lease?

Is there recycling? Presumably you want your service to be as "green" as possible. So is there a way to separate recyclable paper, cans, and so on from the regular garbage?

Check out your prospective neighbors from the lobby directory. Some of your referrals may come from other tenants out of sheer convenience and familiarity. Are there possible referral sources in the building? Some of the best neighbors to have are physicians in family practice. You won't get many referrals from dentists, X-ray centers, urologists, or import-export firms. What about the other neighbors? Do they make the building look successful and professional, or do they seem seedy and downscale? A colleague of mine discovered too late that he had moved into a building with a massage parlor (of the "happy ending" variety) on the ground floor—this was not a catastrophe, but it didn't suit the image he was trying to project to clients.

Qualities of the Suite

Now let's go into the suite. There are a number of aspects you want to consider.

How big is it? You want the overall suite to be big enough to accommodate you and your colleagues (if any), but not so big that you will struggle to make rent. Is there a place for your assistant to work? If not, is the waiting area big enough to put in a reception desk?

How big is the waiting room? You don't need a waiting room as large as one in a medical suite, because therapists seldom have more than one or two people waiting at a time. If, on the other hand, you want to use your waiting room as a group space in the evenings, or for your assistant and a desk, the area will need to be somewhat larger. Also notice where the natural placement of chairs would be. Ideally, you don't want your next client sitting directly outside your door, or departing clients will worry that they may have been overheard. The closer the waiting-room chairs are to therapy-room doors, the more vital soundproofing becomes.

How big should your office be? If you conduct individual therapy, you want a space that will comfortably accommodate all the usual office furniture, plus at least three chairs: one for you, one for your client, and a spare. The spare is for the occasional visitor (a rehabilitation coordinator, spouse, parent, or child) or for the invisible third person your client discusses. Everyone should have enough room to sit without feeling cramped—even the ghosts in the room. If you plan to conduct couples counseling or family therapy, then obviously your room will need to be bigger still.

Look at the suite entry door and locks. Is the door solid? Are the locks sufficient, or would they need to be upgraded? Knock on the walls between the hallway and the suite. Do they sound hollow or solid? Sometimes only drywall separates your suite from the hall. If thieves can't get past your dead bolt, they can simply pound through the drywall and reach around to unlock your door.

Look at the interior doors. Are they solid or hollow core? The latter kind lets through more sound and has a cheaper feel. Will the landlord replace doors in order to rent the place? How do the doors close? Do they latch properly, or will they blow open every time someone enters your waiting room? Look at the space at the bottom of the doors. If the gap is too wide, it will be hard for you to find sound-dampening attachments that will fit.

Check the heating system. Do you have control over the unit's temperature, or are you at the mercy of the landlord? What kind of heating is it? Hot-water radiators often clank or hiss; has that been a problem? Is the heating turned off through the summer until the tenants complain loudly enough to have it turned on in the fall? What about air conditioning? Again, do you have control?

Check the windows. Double-glazed windows will screen out sound more effectively and provide a better temperature buffer in extreme weather. Do the windows open? They don't in most office buildings, so this shouldn't be a deal breaker, but it can be nice to be able to get fresh air into your office.

Look at the exterior windowsills. Are they wide enough for birds to roost outside your windows? This will be cute for about four and a half seconds but will then become distracting for both you and your clients. If birds could roost there, check to see whether there are bird-repellent measures, such as rows of plastic spikes or a gel strip. Also look to see if the sill is solid or made of tin flashing. Rain can sound incredibly loud on tin flashing during intense storms—loud enough to drown out your therapy sessions.

Check the soundproofing. Get a friend to go into each office and talk loudly. Agents hoping to rent the unit may just whisper during this test, so get someone who is on your side. The sound leakage will be greater than when you have furnishings installed, but this should give you some idea of how much sound dampening there is between rooms. In many office buildings, there is nothing but drywall between interior offices.

Check above the ceiling tiles. Most office walls go only as high as the dropped ceiling, not all the way up to the next floor slab. Push up a tile near the wall that divides the suite from the hall or the next suite, and look over. If the wall doesn't go all the way up, then all thieves need to do is go through the space over your walls to get into your suite. Push up a tile near an interior wall (between the office and waiting area, for example). If you can see into the space above the next room, this gap will transmit sound from one room to another. You can reduce this by stuffing insulation into the gap above the wall and extending it a foot or two over the tiles on either side of the wall. Ask your building manager to do this, because you don't want to create a fire hazard.

Does the suite have a sink? You really don't need a washroom if there's one in the hall, but a sink can be a nice feature. You can make tea without having to schlep out to the washroom, you can wash your hands after seeing your flu-laden clients, you can clean up coffee spills more easily, you can wash cups and lunch dishes, and you can do some of your own housekeeping if the cleaners are slack.

What exactly does the building's cleaning involve? Some building maintenance teams are reasonably fastidious, while others simply empty the trash and vacuum occasionally. Is shampooing the carpets included? What if a spill makes carpet cleaning more urgent? Is inside window washing included? What about dusting or vacuuming the windowsills or radiator units?

Come Back Later to Spy on the Property Manager

Thank the agent, head out the door, and go for coffee. Then come back half an hour later and pop into one or two businesses in the building. Talk to someone who won't benefit directly from getting you to rent a suite. Here's what to ask:

- When you have a problem in the building, how responsive is the property manager?

- How satisfied are you with the quality of the cleaning service?

- How well maintained are the common areas? Does the manager change lights, repair elevators, and clean up garbage promptly?

- Have there been any insect or other pest problems in the building that you know of?

- How are the heating and air conditioning systems? Do the controls work properly? Do you have to complain to get the heat turned on in the winter or the air conditioning in the summer?

- Are there any noise problems in the building?

- How do you like the other tenants? Any difficulties there?
- Have there been any unexpected fees or increases? Is there anything I should budget for?

The Lease

Your lease will probably include two main items: the rental rate and the maintenance fee. The rent is often expressed as an amount per square foot per year. Ask about the number of square feet to which the fee is applied. Sometimes it will be the size of the unit alone. More often it will include a portion of the common space in the building: hallways, washrooms, and lobby. So you will pay for more area than is actually inside your door. (On the positive side, this confers a sense of justification if and when you complain to the building manager about the upkeep of the common areas.)

Knowing your annual cost per square foot allows you to compare the cost of buildings in the neighborhood (though make sure you compare maintenance fees as well). To convert it for budgeting, multiply the figure by the actual square footage charged, then divide by twelve. This will give you the monthly rent. Again, don't forget the maintenance fee, which may equal or exceed the rental amount, and all applicable taxes. You want the complete amount of the monthly check you will have to send off to the management company.

What does the rent plus maintenance include? Ask the agent, and be sure to verify the agent's responses when you look at the lease itself. Generally it will include heat, light, water (if the suite is plumbed), exterior window washing (ask how often this is done), pest control (if necessary), building lighting replacements, and general repairs.

Make careful note of all deficiencies in the unit: carpet stains, ceiling tile problems, cracks or poor seals on the windows, marks or nail holes in the walls, missing or broken plates around the light switches and electrical outlets, problems with the radiators or heating system, leaks around the plumbing, and so on. Also create a list of the changes you would want to make to bring the suite up to standard for seeing clients: soundproofing, door replacement, moving the walls, carpet replacement, painting, and anything else that might reasonably be the landlord's responsibility.

Go over your deficiency and wish lists with the agent before you ask her to draw up a lease, and clearly state that you are still looking at other buildings. If the agent senses that the sale has already been made, there will be no motivation to sweeten the pot.

What is the term of the lease? Generally office leases cover more than one year. Consider your own requirements. Are you confident that you want to be locked in for the duration of the proposed lease (which may be three to five years or more)? Is the rental rate fixed for the entire duration of the lease? (Generally it is, though the maintenance fee may fluctuate.) One common arrangement is for a lease to specify the duration (say, two years), plus an option to renew for additional years when that time runs out. If you exercise your right to renew, does the rental rate have to be renegotiated? Generally it does. If you are potentially interested in the unit but want a shorter time commitment or a longer right to renew, say so. These things are usually negotiable.

What if you outgrow your space? If your business expands and there are larger vacant units in the building, is the landlord open to your moving under the terms of your existing lease? Usually the landlord will not want to commit to this in advance, but it can help if you raise the issue when first negotiating for your space.

There. Those are some of the considerations involved in structuring your practice and finding an office. The list is far from complete, however. There will always be unexpected challenges, and any place you settle on will turn out to have deficiencies you didn't think to investigate initially. C'est la vie.

CHAPTER 3

Setting the Scene: The Office as Stage

A mentor of mine used to say that psychotherapy is the ultimate in low-capital-investment professions: all we need are two chairs and a box of tissues. He was right, really.

But when your first client walks through the door, you'll look fairly silly sitting on a camp chair in a bare office. You'll want to give your best performance, and a performer often benefits from the characteristics of the stage. So let's create your space from the walls inward. We'll assume you have opted to buy or lease an unfurnished suite and are starting from scratch. What do you need to do with the space? What do you have to buy? What furnishings do you need to make it functional? Then, once the office itself is ready, how do we furnish *you* so that you look as if you belong there?

PREPARING THE SPACE

You start out with an empty box for an office, but even the box isn't ready. So before you rush off to the store, let's prepare the container. I've signaled some of what you need in the previous chapter, but let's make it explicit.

Soundproofing

Any office seems alarmingly transparent to sound when it's empty. Once you add your furniture, books, and other materials, some of the sound will be absorbed or muffled. You can generally tell, however, if your office is going to need work. As we discussed in the preceding chapter, you might be able to get the sound-dampening work included as part of the deal. Here are some changes to consider.

Fill the walls. Many office-partition walls are simply two sheets of wallboard separated by studs and air. If you are ambitious, you can dampen sound transmission by taking one side off and filling the spaces with special sound-dampening insulation. Then replace the wallboard with a denser sound-deadening brand. Another option is to use injectable foam, which mostly preserves the walls but still involves patching and repainting.

Insulate the ceiling. Office walls often go only as high as the ceiling tiles. Above that is common air space for vents, wiring, and so on. Sound can travel up through the ceiling tiles, over the top of the wall, and down into the next room. Piling fireproof insulation above the wall to the next floor slab, and outward on either side by one to two feet, can significantly reduce sound leakage.

Replace doors. Hollow doors dampen sound less than solid ones. Many offices are furnished with very flimsy (that is, cheap) interior doors or doors with window panels unsuited to a counselor's privacy requirements. Consider replacing them with heavier or sound-insulated versions.

Setting the Scene: The Office as Stage

Insulate doorjambs. Peel-and-stick weatherproofing can reduce sound transmission around the sides and tops of doors, particularly ones that don't close firmly. A door-bottom seal, or sweep seal, can be installed on the door to reduce the gap between the door and the floor. Some of these methods work best if you also install a threshold strip on the floor. Most have rubber strips along the bottom that either sweep across the floor or drop when the door is closed.

Place a white-noise generator in your waiting room. Coupled with a sound system that plays pleasant music, a white-noise generator will obscure sounds coming from the therapy offices in your unit. A purifying air filter can perform double duty by generating white noise, and the variable fan speed is an effective volume control.

Floors, Walls, Windows, Ceilings

Bare floors transmit sound and can create an echoey, hollow feeling in a room. As well, most office suites are not graced with beautiful flooring. Consequently, carpeting is generally a requirement, and wall-to-wall carpet is the most effective at creating a still, sound-dampened environment.

Carpeting should not be a particularly difficult choice. You are not looking for great beauty or deep pile. Its main functions are to dampen sound, provide a sense of warmth and comfort, hide dirt, repel stains, and not attract undue attention. Do not overspend. Imagine people wiping their boots and spilling coffee on it. If this makes you shiver, you are looking at something too fancy.

You should probably select the color of your walls around the same time as that of the carpet, because you don't want them at odds with each other. Pick something neutral and warm. You can always dress it up with artwork and bookshelves. Avoid stark whites, which make a room feel cold and uninviting. Think carefully if you're tempted to choose an idiosyncratic color. Will you want to spend a good part of your life looking at it? Is the choice meant to be a reflection of your personality? Remember that the function of the practice and the room is to serve your clients' needs, not your own.

Even if your building has mirrored windows, clients can feel exposed when they describe deeply personal issues, if they sense that anyone who happens to hang glide by could see them. Blinds and curtains can help create a safer, more relaxed atmosphere. If your unit comes with window coverings, look at them closely: nothing says squalor more loudly than dirty, damaged, or lopsided blinds.

Though seldom looked at directly, ceilings can set the tone for your room. Ragged, mismatched, faded, or stained ceiling tiles should be replaced. If you are doing a major ceiling refit, consider getting rid of any fluorescent-tube lighting and replacing it with recessed or pot lights.

SET DRESSING

Once you've dealt with the bare bones of the suite, it's time to set the stage for your work. Keep in mind that office furnishings get a lot of wear and tear, and that your primary goal is comfort. I once knew a therapist whose office was furnished with excruciatingly delicate antiques that made visitors feel frightened to sit down. I've known others whose stained, worn chairs would make any client wish for a drop cloth or a can of disinfectant. Clients should feel neither repelled by the shabbiness nor frightened by the daintiness of your office. (You'll find an "Office Preparation Sheet" at the websites noted in the introduction.)

Furniture

A lot will happen in your office, so you don't need to perk things up with overdesigned furnishings. Some people shudder at the thought of IKEA, but the Swedish giant has unquestionably furnished more clinical offices (including my own) than any other company. Other options include secondhand-furniture stores and online classified

Setting the Scene: The Office as Stage

sites. You can economize at start-up with some reliable, sturdy furniture, and then replace pieces as your budget permits. Few clients will criticize you for your lack of design élan; generally they have more important things to think about. Here's a short list of what you need:

- *Desks:* Leave the big power desks off your shopping list. Your desk should be subtle and placed out of the way, against a wall or window, freeing most of the space for the client, rather than staking out your private realm. Some people prefer to eliminate desks altogether from therapy spaces, but most cannot manage without.

- *Client chairs:* You want comfort, not just style. Consider all possible sizes and shapes of client. Consider having two types of chair so clients have a choice—a comfortable wingback or tub chair and a padded, straight-backed model. If the latter matches your waiting-room seating, you can swap them around.

- *Your chair:* You will spend far more time sitting in your office than any client will, so spend more on your chair and take the time to ensure that it suits you ergonomically. Don't go for the executive power chair. Hide the money in good engineering and comfort that's carefully chosen to fit your own body shape. You want the height to be adjustable so that you can raise or lower yourself to the client's eye level.

- *Bookshelves:* Built-in shelving is lovely, but it's not practical for many office suites and can't be moved around if you change your mind. Waist-high shelving frees wall space for art, certificates, and a whiteboard. If you do need to get tall units, be sure they are anchored properly to the walls (particularly if you live in earthquake country).

- *File cabinets:* Front-loading (vertical) cabinets project awkwardly into a room but can work when placed next to a desk or in the corner between your desk and the wall. A lateral cabinet will free up more of your floor space (and can be placed in your waiting area if it is bigger than you need). You will want all cabinets to be lockable so they can be used for confidential records. Resist the temptation to buy the cheapest available, or the drawers will exact a price from your well-being forever after.

- *Lamps:* Standard office fluorescent lighting is never calming. Leave it off, and substitute with floor, table, and desk lamps. If you use compact fluorescents, buy the variety that casts a warmer light. Always be sure to stock extras of every type of bulb you use.

- *Coffee or side tables:* You will want one or more low tables for your waiting room. You may also want some kind of table next to the client's chair in the consulting room for tissues, notebooks, cups, and any handouts or forms you provide. Get something you don't have to place between you and the client, because this imposes a psychological barrier.

- *Storage unit:* You will want to have a stash of extra pens, writing pads, tissues, and dozens of other supplies, so some form of storage is essential. There may be a cabinet built into the suite, but if not, you will need a freestanding one. If it closes and is attractive enough, you can place it in your waiting area.

A Whiteboard or Flip Chart

No matter what type of therapy or coaching you practice, you will discuss complex issues with your clients. Some clients will learn vastly better if you can give them a visual representation to consult. Hence a whiteboard or flip chart can be an invaluable tool.

Almost every session with a client can present opportunities for presenting visual material: graphs of mood changes, lists of emotion-related words, diagrams of the sequence of distress, models of communication patterns, family trees, identification of thoughts preceding negative emotions, pros and cons of various options in decision making—the possibilities are endless. Once you write something on the board, you can leave it there for the rest of the session for reference.

As well, both anxiety and depression disrupt concentration and memory. Clients may look at us, apparently rapt, but almost always, their attention is flickering to us and away, off to the troubling future and back to the regrettable past. When they return to the room, it often takes them a moment to remember what's going on. "Where were we? Oh yes,…" Having something on the whiteboard can help them stay on track and reorient themselves when they momentarily derail.

There are downsides to a basic whiteboard. Sometimes you'll use it with a client to list the qualities of a good life, the thoughts that inspire suicidal feelings, the good reasons not to get well, the evidence for and against a self-perception of worthlessness. Then the session ends. You'll want to make a note of the more salient points, but you'll be rushed for time and your next client will be waiting. Or you'll want to go back to the topic during the next appointment, but you don't want to have to re-transcribe everything onto the board. Or you'll want to send the notes home with the client.

One alternative, if money is no object, is an electronic whiteboard that enables you to create a paper copy. Unfortunately, technology often seems to get in the way of human contact. A low-cost alternative is simply to use a flip chart.

At the end of the session, it's a good practice to flip the page over or pick up the eraser when you stand up. This effectively communicates that the client's private information will be removed before the next person comes in. You should also ensure that the flip chart or whiteboard is blank before every new session. Even if you have been doing research-related work or running a clinic committee meeting, clients may think that anything on the board is someone else's private information. This will cause them to worry that their own information will be treated just as informally, making them more reluctant to open up.

Degrees and Qualifications

Medical specialists often have a wall plastered with degrees, awards, and certificates, which can give them an air of tremendous authority and dignity, as well as provide a whopping placebo effect to their patients (which is all to the good). The sheer profusion of qualifications can be intimidating, however. Clients in therapy or coaching situations want to know they are speaking with a trained professional, but you want to join with them in the effort rather than bludgeon them with your expertise. To avoid the "wall of intimidation" effect:

Don't post every qualification you have. If you have two degrees in one field (such as a master's degree and a Ph.D. in psychology), just hang the more advanced degree. If you have degrees in different fields but both relate to your current work (for example, you are an executive coach with a Ph.D. in psychology and a master's degree in business administration), hang them both up.

Limit the certificates to between two and four. Beyond four, the wall begins to look like a lawyer's office. Post only significant items, like your license to practice and any major awards you have received. Don't put up certificates from continuing-education workshops or thank-you notes from sponsors of your talks.

Don't throw your qualifications in the client's face. Avoid hanging the certificates so that they are directly in front of people when they are sitting in the client chair. Take special pains to avoid the "halo effect," in which a person looking at you from that chair will see you framed by your precious qualifications.

Split up the certificates. Rather than hang them all in one place, scatter them around the room and intersperse them with artwork. This creates a more subtle effect.

Clocks

In a physician's office, a clock is unnecessary—both patient and physician know the visit will last only a few minutes. In your own office, time passes more slowly. Most clinicians operate on a fifty-minute hour, and few of us can gauge that length of time with any accuracy. Clients won't know whether they have time to bring up that one last topic, and you won't know when to bring the session to a close. Consequently, a clock is a necessity.

You need one clock that is clearly visible to the client. It's best if this is a rather small and unobtrusive analog model that sweeps gently along rather than attracting attention each time the numbers change. Avoid pointing the clock directly at the client's chair, where it will psychically shout, "Hurry up and get out!" Off to one side is better, where it will simply purr "Don't bother about me; I'm here if you want me."

You need to know the time too, and a clock placed for the client can be hard for you to see unless you obviously glance in that direction, which is as bad as looking at your watch. Innocent though it may be, some clients will always interpret this as meaning, "I'm bored and can't wait for this to be over." So you may find it helpful to have a second clock placed discreetly on a shelf somewhere behind the client, where you can glance at it without the client's noticing, thus avoiding anxieties about your level of interest.

The Client's View

Sit in your client's chair and look around the room. Hallucinate a silhouette of yourself into your usual chair and see what surrounds it. What may seem to you to be a solitary bit of clutter neatly placed off to one side may turn out to be directly in the client's field of vision, just past your left shoulder. Make a point of scanning the entire room at eye level, and see what jumps out at you.

A colleague of mine tried this and realized to her dismay that all of her books on avoiding professional burnout, *Handling the Difficult Client*, and so on were placed directly in the client's field of view. Another noticed that she had inadvertently collected all of her books on sex and sexuality there, potentially implying that it was the only thing she read about or treated.

Look at your own bookshelf from the client's position. Notice where your eye naturally falls. These are the most salient shelves. Banish books that imply you are having significant problems yourself (*Avoiding Burnout, The Wounded Healer*), your introductory psychology textbooks, the trashy novels you secretly read at lunch, the books on handling problem clients, the self-help books you wouldn't recommend to your worst enemy, and all books on managing the finances of your private practice (including this book). Shift those books upward or downward, and replace them with scholarly books on your specialty areas of practice, books on diversity, a book or two on sexuality (this subtly gives clients permission to put such issues on the table), the self-help books you most frequently recommend, high-level books on practice and therapy, and other books that communicate your expertise, interests, and breadth of knowledge.

Look for other obvious problems. The tangle of wires under your desk may be invisible to you, but perhaps it is right in your client's field of view. The stack of papers on the sideboard may seem innocuous, but to the client it shouts disorganization. You may have resigned yourself to a picture frame that never seems to hang straight, but your client may find it unbearably distracting.

Your Waiting Room

The Disney theme parks have an interesting design idea: make waiting in line part of the ride. They furnish waiting areas with things to look at, signs to read, and even guides and actors entertaining the crowd. It's a good practice to design your clinic the same way. The function of the waiting room is to allow clients to set aside their immediate concerns ("What shall I make for dinner?") and prepare to examine deeper elements of their lives.

- *Furniture alignment:* You want to enhance the sense of privacy for all clients. If you have lots of chairs, orient magazines and other elements of the space toward the ones farthest from the inner consulting-room doors.

- *Sound:* As mentioned earlier, an air purifier will help to obscure voices in adjoining offices. Supplement this with an MP3 player or radio and reasonably good speakers. Soothing music will do much more to prepare your client for the work than will an all-news or talk radio station.

- *Water:* Clients often arrive in a rush, experience anxiety about the upcoming session, and talk more in session than they may at any other time. For all of these reasons, it can be useful to have a source of pure drinking water for them. If the water cooler is in the waiting room, it will be accessible to everyone in the clinic.

- *Washroom keys:* Many office buildings have locked washrooms. Have the keys available and obvious in the waiting area (perhaps with a sign and directions) so that clients don't have to ask your assistant for them. Attach a fob large enough that the key won't be placed in someone's pocket and forgotten.

- *Coatrack:* Many clients will arrive wearing a coat. If you don't provide a coatrack, they will either leave the coat on (giving the visit a rushed, tentative feeling) or lay it over your empty chair (eliminating it as a prop for absent spouses, bosses, children, deceased family members, alternative points of view, and so on). A coatrack also affords you a handy bit of "therapy business": you can offer to take and hang up the client's coat, subtly but effectively demonstrating care for the client. If your waiting room is unattended, the coatrack is better placed inside the consulting room.

- *Magazines:* You can stock your waiting area with whatever is most popular or offers the cheapest subscription, but these magazines may provide messages that clash with your interventions. News magazines focus on catastrophes, fashion magazines emphasize unrealistic body weight and the ephemeral, design magazines suggest the importance of status, and many health care magazines encourage hypochondriasis. Ensure that your magazines are interesting and fit your service. Some options include books outlining local hikes and walks, publications about healthy diets (such as the *Nutrition Action Health Letter*), a magazine about psychology that doesn't trivialize the subject (*Scientific American Mind* is a reasonable choice), and magazines about local travel or the outdoors (for example, *National Geographic*). The goal is to make the waiting room a positive and helpful aspect of the experience rather than simply a place to "kill time."

- *Exterior signage:* It takes time for many management companies to update hallway door signs and lobby directories. Get this started as soon as possible. New clients often know the building they are looking for, but they assume they will be able to get the suite number from the directory. If you're not listed, this creates a negative first impression.

- *Interior signage:* Unless you have a large practice and employ a full-time assistant, your waiting room will often be unattended. To ensure that clients (and delivery people) don't pound on the consulting-room door when you are in session, put up sliders on each interior door that flip from "Available" or "Vacant" to "Occupied" or "In Session." You might also consider posting one or two tastefully designed signs to address relevant issues: "If no one is here to greet you, please have a seat and a clinician will be with you shortly." "Please turn off cell phones during appointments."

PROPS AND TOOLS

Now the office looks quite a lot like an office, but we're still missing the props: the objects you or your assistant will need to keep the place running. Add these and you're nearly there.

Stationery

Your business will benefit from having a visual identity. Once you have settled on a name, you will want a logo, font, color scheme, or, more likely, all three so that your communications are immediately identifiable as being from you. Their design will seem easy: you've been working with fonts and colors all your life; surely you can come up with your own layout and logo. Perhaps. But unless you have significant design experience, working with a graphic designer will help. You'll regret it when you first pay the person, but you'll be glad of it from then on. Be sure to get electronic versions of your logo in various file formats and resolutions, in both color and gray scale (something that will print nicely when you don't want to pay for color).

Once you have a logo and a design, it's time to look for a reliable and inexpensive printer. If you use an established company, you won't have to go through the hassle of finding and sending your files to a new printing services company every year or two. What to get?

- *Business cards:* You want something that looks professional, so avoid making your own. Check the price breaks by quantity: it's easy for a printer to create more copies once everything is set up, so the per-card price usually drops by more than half as you order larger numbers. If your information might change or you have multiple providers, you can often get the color portion made up as blanks in large quantities and then have the black-and-white name and contact information added later.

- *Letterhead:* Your letterhead should be crisp and professional, so avoid overdesigning it. You'll use letterhead for dozens of tasks, so don't skimp on quantity.

- *Brochures:* We'll talk more about brochure design in chapter 4. Depending on your budget, you may want a full-color or black-and-white version. If you get black-and-white, your grayscale logo will come in handy. You can dress it up a bit by having it printed on tinted paper.

- *Electronic letterhead:* In addition to your printed stationery, you will want a word-processing file that incorporates your logo and contact information as letterhead. You can use this as a template from which to generate your bills, various forms, and so on, enabling you to print hard copies without having to put letterhead in your printer.

Electronics

You'll want a computer, of course, and perhaps one for an assistant. There's no need to go high-end, because most of the work in your office will be fairly standard word-processing and spreadsheet work. A laptop will relieve you of the need to have home and office computers with the inevitable shuttling of files back and forth, and you can use it for presentations. What else?

- *A phone system:* Arrange this early, because there might be more of a delay in installation than you anticipate. Consider whether you want more than one line or voice mailbox, and purchase phones with your choice in mind.

Setting the Scene: The Office as Stage

- *Wireless broadband:* You don't want to fiddle with wires every time you change rooms, and wireless Internet is relatively simple to set up. Your wireless access point should have *WPA* (Wi-Fi protected access) encryption or better. Give your *SSID* (service set identifier, the name your wireless access point is broadcasting) a name that doesn't identify your clinic (to discourage potential hackers).

- *Printers/fax machines:* You'll find that having a copier-printer in each room is extremely handy. The one in your assistant's area should also have fax capability. Faxes are fading a bit in popularity but remain essential for the time being. Rather than buy a dedicated fax line that will go unused most of the time, consider piggybacking a second ring tone onto your regular line.

- *Calculators:* Yes, your computer has a calculator built in, but you will seldom regret having a separate calculator in every room.

- *Point-of-sale terminal:* Some clients will pay cash, but this entails trips to the bank and having secure storage in your suite. You can accept checks, but fewer and fewer people use them. Accepting credit cards will be a great convenience for many of your clients, though you will want to pressure your bank for the lowest possible deposit fees (being a health care professional often helps). Debit cards are best of all: easy for clients, reasonably low fees for you, and instant deposit. A simple device that runs on your broadband should do nicely.

Coaches and therapists are seldom technologically savvy, so setting up the electronic side of your business can seem daunting. Keep in mind that all of these devices are meant for the general public to understand them, though paying a technophile to do the job may save you hours that would be better spent on other tasks.

67

THE COSTUME DEPARTMENT

Much is made of the need for honesty and transparency in the relationship between clinician and client. This is undeniably useful, but the candor is inevitably selective. Some mornings you would rather be home in bed, some hours you are uncomfortably aware that you should have gone to the washroom before the appointment began, and with some clients, you go through periods of feeling lost and uncertain about what to do next.

Like it or not, the clinician role is just that: a role. Hopefully, it is a role through which your personality and genuine style will be able to shine, but just as actors must set aside their own lives and take up the mantle of a role when they walk onto a stage, therapists must be able to set aside their own concerns for a time and create an environment in which clients can be comfortable and cared for. Part of this process involves dressing to convey your intention.

Clothing Tips

How should you dress? Much depends on your personal style, but remember that your clothing communicates. It's worthwhile to ask yourself just what your shirt is saying to your clients. In researching this book, I asked fellow clinicians for useful tips. Here are the resulting suggestions (with a few of my own thrown in). If some of the comments seem contradictory, the art is to look for the golden mean, or for what works for you.

Dress your age, but backwards. If you look very young, dressing a bit more formally and conservatively than you normally would can help make you look more experienced. As you get older, you can appear somewhat authoritative, and there is more room to dress down. Clothes that might help elevate a twenty-five-year-old into the "health professional" role might elevate a sixty-year-old to the "imposing banker" look, which should be avoided.

Setting the Scene: The Office as Stage

Don't overdress. The woman's power suit and the businessman's suit and tie look dressy, but they impose too much of a mask over most therapists' appearance, communicating superiority, formality, impatience, and possibly an interest in money over compassion. This can alienate clients rather than help them to feel at ease. Consequently, most therapists avoid formal business dress for their clinic days.

There is a basic minimum. No matter how old or imposing you are, your clothing should be neat and clean. In most settings and with most populations, you should avoid jeans. Excessive informality can suggest to clients that you will be equally casual about your records, your technique, or confidentiality. Clients entrust the therapist with a great deal, and it is important that you look (as well as be) fully deserving of that trust.

Dress for the function. A neat but informal appearance is typically valued for therapy. When you appear in court, however, you should dress much more formally, with a conservative business suit (for men and women). This may not be your usual look, but settings like this are more about communicating competence than expressing yourself.

Dress to match your clientele. If you work as an executive coach, you will typically find it most helpful to dress like an executive. It will be hard to convince a corporate vice president that your ideas can help him make a good impression if you look more like a mailroom attendant. If you see more working-class clients, you will want to dress somewhat more like them. The intent is to join with your clients, not intimidate them. If you routinely notice that most of your clients dress better than you do, step it up a notch. If they dress a bit more informally, this is fine: you're at work and they're not.

> *Dress in a way that truly and accurately portrays who you are. If your values and lifestyle are sort of hippieish, wear sandals and Indian skirts to work. If you're a corporate type, don suits, designer labels, and expensive shoes. We sell not only our skills but also ourselves as a*

> *product. The ways we present ourselves will give clients a good idea about our values, approaches, and lifestyles.*

Don't shout with your clothing. In the same way that you wouldn't want to tower over your clients or drown them out with your voice, you don't want your clothing to distract from the work.

> *It seems to me that any clothing in good taste is okay, but whereas it's fine for it to be almost anywhere on the scales of expensive and not, trendy and not, and so on, it needs to be sufficiently unobtrusive as to not draw too much attention to the therapist per se. The therapist's personality need not take center stage, and clothing is an important aspect of that.*

Be comfortable. Therapy can be exhausting work, and one way to stay fresh is to wear clothing in which you feel comfortable.

> *I find that few clients actually care. I recall a whole day of wearing mismatched socks and realizing that nobody noticed. I find that either clients are too involved in their own issues to care what you wear, or when they need to project onto you, then whatever you wear, do, or say can be a source of suspicion, criticism, or admiration. Be respectful and comfortable in your skin. If I have to sit there the whole day, I do not wear tight pants or uncomfortable shoes.*

Be stylish, not fashionable. Whereas many of us regard style and fashion as synonyms, English expatriate Quentin Crisp argues in *Doing It with Style* (1981) that they are opposites. Fashion involves trying to look like everyone else, eliminating your uniqueness. Style involves finding what makes you unique and moving it to the forefront. Crisp wrote that human uniqueness is rapidly becoming undervalued and most people are engaged in a headlong rush toward blandness.

> *I found purple hair a really fun thing for little kids in my practice.... Whatever a therapist wears needs to be worn*

> with confidence. However, suit jackets with naked women
> on the lining, tight blue jeans that show off more than the
> money in your pocket, and hotpants (which I actually wore
> to a job interview many years ago) and short skirts that
> show off undies, coupled with see-through blouses and so on,
> are not appropriate, since our clients might find themselves
> dealing with our sexual issues rather than their own!

SPECIAL CLOTHING TIPS FOR WOMEN

Alas, the genders are not equal when it comes to clothing and expectations: women have more layers of subtlety available to them, which can be a curse for the therapist attempting to decipher her own semiotics. This is obviously not a topic about which I can claim special expertise, so I asked a group of female clinicians for their suggestions and received a number of replies. Here are some of their tips (for which I take no personal responsibility):

Have no visible cleavage. My advisers inform me that an alarming number of men speak directly to women's breasts (perhaps mistaking them for organs of hearing). This can be distracting in the therapy environment. As well, a therapist usually wants to reduce the potential for clients to believe they are receiving sexual signals from her.

> When I supervised psych assistants at the youth jail, our
> various rules were no spaghetti-strap tank tops, no belly
> shirts that expose the midriff, no flip-flops; and if you have
> a navel piercing or tattoo on your lower back, your client
> shouldn't know about it. Obviously that would apply for the
> various other piercings some of them had elsewhere as well!

Above-the-knee outfits are ill advised. Most therapists will be more comfortable in clothing that enables free movement and leg crossing without excessive caution or an intervening desk or table.

Consider your accessories. As elsewhere, consider the associations that certain accessories or manners of dress may communicate.

> *Some tasteful leather pieces (belts, purses, shoes, other accessories) would generally be appropriate, but avoid leather pants, dresses, skirts, bodysuits, and any corresponding paraphernalia. Yes to tasteful jewelry in moderation, but for example, avoid chains with marijuana leaves or rings that look like skulls (I have seen psychologists wear things like this).*

CLOTHING TIPS FOR MEN

Many men arguably need more advice in the area of clothing than do women. On the other hand, men generally have it easier than women when it comes to dressing, because there are fewer options and clearer expectations (perhaps because many men require absolutely clear guidelines to avoid offending someone).

Here's a reply from a male psychologist that echoes much that has been said previously:

> *It seems clear to me that formal, dark suits with whitish shirts and ties are essential in formal settings like court and other legal situations. However, in the clinic or office, it seems that more-informal clothes are often necessary to create an air of emotional accessibility (that is, clothes that are casual but fairly new and fashionable). It seems necessary to create an appearance of financial success, as an illustration of competence. If I had a general criticism of the dress of male psychologists, it would be that many dress too formally, which can make them appear emotionally remote.*

Here are more suggestions for men:

Button your shirt to a reasonable height. Just as female therapists want to steer away from advertising their cleavage, male therapists should not impose on their clients the sight of their pectorals or chest hair.

No shorts. Most men do not wear shorts well, and bare legs can be a distraction when you are seated directly across from someone. You are a clinician, not a bicycle courier.

Avoid sandals. Almost every therapist sits with legs crossed most of the time, elevating a foot to a position within the client's visual field. If you don't want the client to spend the entire session pondering the state of your calluses, toenails, and arches, wear shoes. Note: socks do not solve the sandal problem; they exacerbate it by calling your judgment into question.

Avoid short socks. Ankle-height athletic socks are great for workouts but not for the office. They may be invisible when you look down at your long pants in the full-length mirror, but they won't be when you cross your legs and display your hairy ankles to the client.

The Olfactory Environment

The sense of smell is closely related to emotion and memory, and you can never tell how a client will react to a particular scent. In general, it's best for therapists to limit the use of scented products, including aftershave, perfume, and even scented deodorant, for a number of reasons:

- *Allergies:* More and more people seem to be allergic to the chemicals used in producing scents, so many health care settings now forbid the use of scented products.

- *Salience:* Since cigarettes were banned from most workplaces and restaurants, many people notice even a hint of smoke. Similarly, as scents become less common, their unexpected presence becomes more noticeable and distracting.

- *Perceptual differences:* A certain product may smell different to different people. Certain colognes that some find quite pleasant smell unnatural and unpleasant to others.

- *Associations:* A light floral scent may remind some clients of springtime outdoors, but to others it will bring to mind oppressive Aunt Hilda and her relentless complaining.

- *Intensity:* A scent that seems innocuous when you put it on can become pervasive and oppressive in a small consulting room over time. You will probably not notice this yourself, because habituation to smells happens within minutes. So if you must use scented products, do so sparingly. I have had the unpleasant task of gently informing young interns that the impenetrable wall of cologne they wore was unacceptable in a work environment, fearing that a spark from electrical equipment might ignite the fume cloud surrounding them and we would all be immolated where we stood.

In sum, any scent may produce either positive or negative associations. Although the positives may be subtle and welcome, the negatives pose a significant problem. The absence of a scent is seldom an issue, however: few people react negatively to a therapist they cannot smell.

What about incense? Again, you don't want clients to be overcome by the scent of an office. If you want to overcome the smells of new furniture, old carpets, or intermittently gassy clinicians, you might consider burning a stick late on Friday afternoons, after the last client has left, allowing the scent to fade over the weekend to just above the threshold of perception. Don't leave while it's still burning, obviously.

※

The walls are soundproof, the rooms are furnished, the electronics are humming quietly, the professional is dressed. Now, where do you get your clients?

CHAPTER 4

Getting Referrals

Clinicians are seldom taught how to promote themselves. If anything, we are taught *not* to do so. Many of us think we should sit behind closed doors and the world will come pounding to be let in. The truth is, your expertise and professionalism may be good reasons for people to come to see you, but they're not the reasons why people will. If you practice in an ethical and effective way, you may do a lot of good, but only if people actually come to see you. Being competent is not enough. You need to strategize.

DEFINE YOUR PRODUCT

Most newspaper ads have one thing in common: they tell you what they're selling. The public announcements of therapists and coaches, on the other hand, tend to be vaguely inspirational: "Become the true self you have always wanted to be." What would you actually get if you went to a therapist who advertised this way? You can't tell.

This reluctance of clinicians to say what they really offer stems from a fear of relinquishing part of the potential market. Every statement you make says what you *don't* do just as much as what you do. Most professionals feel instinctively that they don't want to say anything that would cause someone to try someone else: "I want to get people into my practice, not give them reasons to stay away." This is the equivalent of calling your business Anne's Store instead of Anne's Sofa Bed Store. "But if I say I sell sofa beds, I'll turn off everyone who wants to buy dining-room tables." True, but you don't have dining-room tables to sell, so what's the problem? The people who want a sofa bed *really* want a sofa bed, but they will never show up in your store unless you tell them you have sofa beds.

Before you can get referrals, then, you need to define your business clearly. Take some time to do this on paper (a "Potential Referral Sources" worksheet is available at the websites noted in the introduction to help you with this task). Who are your potential clients in terms of age group, socioeconomic group, language spoken, gender, minority status, or profession? What would they want from you, and what would you offer them? What are your particular specialties, including ones that you share with other providers and ones that might be unique to your practice? Come up with a short list of the problems and issues you see. Don't make it more than four items long, or no one will remember it (and they will think you're trying to do everything). How would such individuals find out about you and ultimately come to see you? Once you've done this, you're ready to consider how to find these people and get some of them into your office.

IDENTIFY YOUR MOST PROMISING REFERRAL SOURCES

It can be tempting to ask, "Where are all the depressed, anxious, bulimic, insert-your-specialty-here clients?" This is a good exercise that may give you some hints about how to promote your practice.

But you don't want, will never have, and could not handle all of those clients. You need to know the whereabouts only of the small subset that will actually show up in your office.

When I opened a private clinic, I tried to get the word out as far and wide as possible, reasoning that if I reached enough professionals, I'd get enough referrals to sustain my practice. In retrospect, the vast majority of people who received my private-practice announcement probably threw it away. The majority of my referrals came from people I already knew: the very people I had neglected most in my notification efforts. I would have been much better off to focus my efforts not on the bulk of the provider population, but on the few professionals most likely to refer: those who knew my work best.

Isn't this limiting? No. Professionals trade the names of people to whom they refer. If you do good work, your name will spread. Your colleagues will become your advertisers.

Take twenty minutes to write down names of people who know you, your work, or your prospective client populations (again, refer to the "Potential Referral Sources" worksheet available at the websites noted in the introduction). If you don't know who the key players are, conduct a search to find out. Be sure you do not miss these individuals in your promotional efforts.

CREATE A PAMPHLET

Your service should have a simple three-panel pamphlet printed on standard letter-sized or A4 paper (other sizes may not fit into standard racks). It is more important to have a pamphlet than to have one that's flawlessly designed. You can always upgrade it later. Write the text of the pamphlet yourself and then create it using desktop publishing software or by hiring someone with a few basic design skills. Some tips:

- Decide whether to print the brochure in full color, gray scale plus one color, or gray scale only (which is cheaper). This will determine some of your design choices. If you opt for gray scale, you can have it printed on tinted paper to liven it up a bit. If you want color, check to see whether having just one side with color content reduces the price.

- Decide whether to create small batches of brochures at your local copy center or have larger numbers made up by an offset printer (which can be much cheaper per copy, particularly if you use color).

- The front panel (when printing, the right-most panel on side A) should have the name of your service (or your own name), your logo (if any), your Web address, and a very brief slogan or description that hints about the type of service you offer. Your service name should be in the upper third of the panel, because many racks only show the upper third of each pamphlet. If you include a photo, make it simple (particularly if you plan to print in gray scale). The photo might be of you, or it could be an attractive picture that somehow complements your service (if you don't have a picture you like, type "stock photo" into an Internet search engine to find companies that sell photos for the purpose).

- The inset panel (visible when you open the front flap; the left-most panel on side A) is a prominent place to put important information, such as how to refer, your contact and location information, or a brief description of the work you do.

- The three panels on the inside of the pamphlet (side B) provide a wide expanse in which to describe your service or the difficulties you most commonly see.

- The rear of the pamphlet (the middle panel of side A) is the least obvious of the six panels. You can leave it blank, place less-important material here, put a brief personal bio here (perhaps with a photo if you haven't put one elsewhere), or list your contact information for the benefit of those who have been "hooked" by your other information.

- Be sure your Web address appears at least once, and preferably twice. The pamphlet is really an invitation to visit your website to learn more about your service.

- Your location information should include all possible methods of contacting you: street address, telephone number, fax number, and e-mail address. Mention the neighborhood or nearest cross street if this is not completely obvious from the address. Consider including a small inset map.

Why do you need a pamphlet? You will include it in mailings to other professionals, display it in your waiting room, offer it to your referral sources, place stacks of them in relevant locations (for example, the Polish neighborhood center if you offer services in Polish), hand it out at every public presentation you give—and you will find myriad other uses as well. A pamphlet is a central part of your promotional efforts.

CREATE A SIMPLE REFERRAL FORM

Your referral sources know that if they are referring someone, they should give you the person's name, contact information, and problem. They'll put all that in the referral note or telephone message. So why do you need a referral form?

You don't. But there are good reasons to have one anyway:

- Offering it gives you a reason to write to your potential referral sources.

- A nice-looking referral form helps your practice look professional.

- A form increases the likelihood that you will receive information you really need (like the client's phone number).

- A form eliminates the need for professionals to write a salutation ("Thank you in advance for seeing this client..."), which saves their time.

- A form helps referral sources remember everything to put down, which makes life easier for them.

- Many professionals have terrible handwriting, so seeing their chicken scratches next to specific items (like "Address:") can help you to decipher them.

- Professionals who keep your form on hand will see your name repeatedly and think of you when they need to refer someone to a therapist.

- If referring professionals get used to your form and your clinic, it will be easier for them to refer to you than to someone else.

- Having a very simple form can communicate that you are easy to work with and don't demand huge amounts of information (read: time) from your referral sources.

What should your form look like? In an ideal world you might include space for every medical test, prescription, and illness the client has ever had: the entire family background, the history of mental health intervention, a complete diagnosis, and so on. But if you demand all this, you will never get a referral. You want potential referral sources to experience relief when they look at your form ("This'll be quick and easy"), not despair ("This'll take me forever, and I'll probably get some of it wrong and look foolish"). So here's what it should look like (a sample is available at the websites noted in the introduction):

- Make it black-and-white for easier copying and faxing.

- Include your own contact information (all modes).

- Make it one page only, full margins, with 12-point or larger type.

- Double-space the lines, or set at one and a half line spaces, leaving plenty of room to write legibly.

- Leave a white block for your source's address stamp.

- Ask the client's gender. Sometimes you can't tell from the name, which makes the initial phone call awkward.

- Don't ask for too much. You can always call your source if you need more information.

- End with a "Comment" block. Give referring professionals some space to write general remarks they think are relevant.

Send your form out with your private-practice announcement, and offer to provide more copies whenever your referral sources need some. Get a printer to make twenty-five-sheet pads of the forms for your frequent referral sources, but have single copies available for most other purposes. Send a single copy with every "Thank you for your referral" note, mentioning that the form is for them to use next time (otherwise they will think you are demanding it for the current client). Have the form on hand by your fax machine, so you can send it at a moment's notice when requested (when professionals ask for one, that means they want to refer someone *now*, not when your assistant gets around to it). Post the referral form on your website in PDF format so people can download and print it.

Remember, you don't really need the referral form. Its function is to make it easier for people to refer to you, not harder. Do not demand it. You want the referral source to feel that the door is open to your clinic and that you will do what it takes to make sure the referral is handled smoothly. You don't want referral sources to feel as if they are filling in an application form that might be rejected.

WRITE AND DISTRIBUTE A PRIVATE-PRACTICE ANNOUNCEMENT

When you open your service, you will want to write a letter of self-introduction, known as the private-practice announcement. Create several versions for various potential referral sources, personalizing each with the recipient's name. Here's what to include (a sample letter is available at the websites noted in the introduction):

- An initial short paragraph announcing the opening of the service.

- The name, location, and all contact information for the service (much or all of this may appear on your letterhead, but you can refer to some or all of it again in the body of the letter). Mention the neighborhood, which may not be obvious from the street address. If the office is close to transit, say so.

- Your short list of specialties, with brief descriptions of each, if necessary.

- A brief description of the services you offer (for example, cognitive behavioral therapy, executive coaching, child custody, and access assessments). Do you handle assessment-only cases? Medicolegal assessments?

- Any particular client populations or areas of special expertise ("In addition, I have particular interest in treating geriatric and sexual minority populations").

- Any languages other than English in which you offer services. (If you provide services only in English, don't bother saying so.)

- Referral options. Can clients self-refer? Do you expect a referral form?

- Client payment options: cash, check, credit card, debit card. Can clients be reimbursed for your services by their health insurance or benefits provider?

- A three-to-four-line description of your training and background, and any special qualifications (such as diplomate status or authorization to perform Workers' Compensation Board assessments).

Enclose a referral form (if you have one), business card, and pamphlet. Send the package to all of your particularly promising referral sources, and tailor each with the person's name and a line or two: "Dear Peter, It was good to see you again at the conference last week. As we discussed over lunch, on June 15 I am opening a new practice…" Once you have done this, create additional packages for your less-promising referral sources (practitioners in the neighborhood, tangential business contacts, specialists who may not know of you), keeping a more formal tone: "Dear Dr. Yuen, I would like to announce that on June 15, I will be opening a new practice…"

Keep a list of everyone you have sent the announcement to, so you don't send anyone the same letter again. When you meet people who might refer clients to you, update the letter and personalize it with their names and send it off to them: "Dear Dr. Singh, in June of this year, my colleagues and I opened a new practice…" Create another version for people who refer to you for the first time without benefit of a prior letter: "Dear Mr. Lang, many thanks for your referral of Jane W. to our service. As you may know, we specialize in…"

REFER TO YOUR OWN REFERRAL SOURCES

Balance theory (Heider, 1958) suggests that human beings instinctively strive for a sense of balance in their relationships. If someone does you a favor, you feel a drive to do something pleasant in return. In the professional world, some forms of balance (like offering payment in exchange for referrals) are appropriately forbidden by most professional organizations. But balance remains relevant. Someone who refers a client to you is implicitly expressing confidence in your abilities. You can feel a desire to be nice to that professional in return, and one way to do so is to refer clients to that person. This can encourage an ongoing pattern of exchange.

Of course, the first priority is the welfare of the client, not the welfare of your practice. If the referral source is unprofessional or incompetent, you might be quite willing to receive clients from that source, but you should avoid referring any clients to that person in return. Refer clients only to professionals who provide excellent care. Fortunately many of your referral sources probably fit the bill. Referring appropriate clients to them serves to maintain and extend these relationships. Perhaps they are in the same line of work as you and refer to you when their own practices are full. If your practice fills, you can return the favor.

Some colleagues provide different services than you do. The local neuropsychologist can refer her anxiety cases to you, and you can refer your head-injury assessments to her. If you get to know the general practitioner who sends clients your way, perhaps you would feel comfortable recommending him to the client seeking a family doctor.

What if you are not sure your referral source sees people with your client's problem? A simple inquiry expresses respect for the professional's work. If the person says anything that leaves you with questions ("I mainly see addictions, but I'm sure I could deal with your client's body dysmorphic disorder"), you don't have to follow up with the referral. Most inquiries along this line don't result in a referral being made, so it won't seem odd to the professional. If you refer the client elsewhere and the professional asks what happened to the referral, you can be candid: "I found out that Marlene Smith sees a lot of body dysmorphic folks in her practice, so I wound up referring him there." This should be accepted without any huffiness, particularly if you follow up by commenting on referrals you would like to make: "I've seen some people with crystal meth problems; do you take those?"

CHOOSE DIRECTORIES WISELY

There are dozens of directory services available for therapists. Placing your name in all of them would be extremely expensive, and most will not pay off with referrals. Which should you pick?

Fewer and fewer people use the yellow pages (preferring instead to search using the Internet), but as of this writing, it is probably still worthwhile to have a listing. It's cheap, easy to arrange, and convenient for anyone who wants to track you down. Very few clients will see you solely due to your listing, but they or your referral sources may know about you and track down your contact information from this source. All you need to list is your name, address, phone number, and website address. Do not bother with a display ad.

Your local professional organization may operate a Web-based referral service. If so, ask listed colleagues how many referrals they get from this source. Some such services are well used; others cost a great deal, but no one ever uses them.

National and international professional organizations sometimes offer referral services as an add-on to the regular membership fee. Very few prospective clients know about these listings, however, and even fellow members are more likely to use a local listing service. Consequently, you may get referrals only from out-of-town professionals looking for a therapist for clients moving to your area—a rare event. Save your money.

Some communities have neighborhood business directories, but few of them are widely used. Unless you have strong evidence otherwise, you can pass up this option.

Some directories are population specific rather than neighborhood specific. If you speak Turkish and there is a local Turkish community directory, it might be worthwhile to place your name in it. Most larger gay communities have a business directory, many of which are widely used. Again, check with colleagues who have listings to get their impressions.

Most large communities also have compilations of all the local social services, including private practitioners. These directories sit on the shelf of almost every service listed therein, and there is usually a Web version as well. It can be very useful to be listed in them, and the cost, if any, is generally minimal.

GET ON AGENCY REFERRAL LISTS

Various organizations keep lists of preferred providers of mental health services. If they recommend you and hear back good things, they are likely to use you more and more often. Here are some possibilities:

- *Local publicly funded clinics:* Public services are usually flooded with referrals and often seek to thin out the waiting list by mentioning the availability of private providers ("If the waiting list is too long and you have the resources, we have the names of some people you could see privately..."). The list is also used when someone does not quite meet the agency's mandate ("We're only able to see people who have been hospitalized..."). Call the local services serving your preferred client population and find out if they have such a list.

- *Clinical trials research groups:* Universities, hospitals, and private companies conduct clinical trials of specific treatments (such as psychoactive medications or various psychotherapies). Generally the volunteers for these studies are screened to see if they meet the inclusion criteria (such as no history of hospitalization, no major medical problems, and so on), and many or most are not accepted. The people doing the screening feel obliged to offer these folks *something*, however, and usually it is a recommendation for a service that may be able to see them. That could be you. Find out who does clinical trials on your approximate client population in your area, and provide them with information on your service.

- *Disability insurers:* Mental health issues are among the most common causes of employment disability claims and may represent a higher cost per disabled employee than most physical causes of disability (Dewa, Chau, & Dermer, 2010). Consequently, disability case managers often refer people to private clinicians to try to help clients return to work. They want to know that the service will be short term and that the provider will use methods supported by the research evidence. If you offer such services, find out who the main insurers are in your area and send them a clear introduction letter (preferably with pamphlets and cards), identifying exactly which client populations you deal with most effectively and how to refer. Don't overstate the breadth of your expertise. If they refer someone with an arcane problem and you don't do well with the client, that'll be your last referral. Go with your strengths.

- *Automobile insurers:* Automobile insurers often arrange and pay for the treatment of people who have been traumatized in auto accidents (or those who need neuropsychological evaluations). If you do this work, it can be useful to have your name on the local insurers' or adjusters' lists.

- *Health maintenance organization (HMO) and preferred provider organization (PPO) panels:* In the United States, many prospective clients are covered by HMOs or PPOs that keep lists (panels) of providers that people can see. It can be difficult to get on these panels. Many insurers have a restricted number of providers and accept new providers only when existing members leave. As well, panel members generally must accept a contracted fee for their services that is often below their usual fee. Nevertheless, provider panels are a huge source of clients for psychologists and other therapists.

- *Human resources departments:* Large organizations often fund private psychotherapy services for their employees, and some human resources departments maintain lists of providers for their employees. Sometimes employees are reimbursed only if they see someone on the list. Call up the HR departments of the large employers in your area. If they have such a list, see if you can be added to it.

CREATE A REFERRAL NETWORK

Most private practitioners have their own lists of colleagues to whom they refer, and most bemoan the inadequacy of their lists. Even people who have been practicing for years often have few ideas about whom to refer to for early psychosis, neuropsychological testing, or even their own specialties when their practices are full. You could be the solution to this problem and, at the same time, enhance your own referral rate.

Invite a group of colleagues to exchange information in order to create a good referral network among yourselves. There are many ways to do this, but for all of them, you want to specify the types of information everyone should provide to the group:

- Name
- Address
- Contact information
- Credentials
- Populations seen
- Services offered (including therapeutic modality)
- Languages spoken

The entire process can be carried out by e-mail. Create a form, send it out for people to fill in the relevant information, and get them to send it back to you. Compile the forms into a single document (or have an assistant do so) and distribute the result to the list.

You could also run a face-to-face business networking event. Set up the meeting, preferably in a setting where everyone can mingle. Encourage everyone to bring either a stack of their pamphlets or copies of a completed form, like the one described previously. Provide name tags. Impose assignments to help overcome shyness ("Your job is to talk to at least six people you don't know and exchange information about your practice").

To make this activity more tightly structured, consider running it like speed dating. Create a circle of pairs around the room and have people pick one of two roles (for example, blue or green). Give the "blues" three minutes to describe their practices, and then the "greens." Have everyone exchange pamphlets or forms. Then have the "greens" move one person to the left and start again. With large numbers you can use trios (one sits still, one moves clockwise, one counterclockwise). With smaller numbers, appoint one individual to trade roles (for example, green becomes blue) with each person he meets; this will allow each person to meet everyone else in the room. This exercise can be fun, quick, and productive, and it forces the shy to take part. Just one evening like this could build your own list significantly.

Would your serious colleagues really go for such an exercise? I wondered that myself, so I volunteered to try it out at a professional meeting. One of the association staff remarked, "I've never seen most of those people smile before." Go figure.

Why should this be up to you? The secret is that by virtue of organizing the list or event, you will be more remembered than anyone else who takes part. Just ensure that you aren't forced to sit things out. If you run a speed networking session, get someone else to be the timekeeper.

KEEP A REFERRAL BOOK

You'll never remember everyone to whom you might send referrals or everyone who refers clients to you, so don't try. Keep a referral book.

One section is for people to whom you refer clients, a page for each. Attach the clinician's card, pamphlet, or other information to the page. Make note of the referrals you make and any information on the outcomes of the cases. If clients report back that the service was poor, you can avoid sending that professional referrals in the future. You can also keep a list of people to whom you will *never* refer clients.

The other half of the book should contain a page for every professional who refers clients to you. Note the referrals you receive and how the cases work out, and keep track of thank-you notes or practice updates you send. If they routinely refer inappropriate clients, if they sabotage your work by referring clients to other resources while you are seeing them, or if they are pushy or difficult to deal with, make a note.

Once you've had a book like this for a while, it becomes quite useful. You can use it when you need to make a referral, and you know which referral sources you want to thank or cultivate. Another option, of course, is to keep a referral spreadsheet with this information.

RETURN REFERRAL CALLS PROMPTLY!

Someone calls you about a possible referral. You're in session and your assistant is out, so the caller leaves a voice-mail message. What happens?

Just as drugs and radiation have half-lives, so too do referral calls. There is a certain length of time after which an inquiry is only half as likely to result in an actual client appointment being booked. No one knows the half-life of a referral call, but a colleague of mine swears it's about three hours. She's probably right.

Clients generally call in when they have worked up their courage and are ready to make the leap and book an appointment. They usually have more than one provider's name on hand. If you don't call them back quickly, either they will call the next person on the list or they might lose their nerve (*Maybe I don't really need this, Maybe I can stand it a bit longer, Maybe I don't really want to discuss my problems with a stranger*).

Professionals who call on behalf of their clients are busy. An unfinished phone call sits as an open file in their minds or on their desks. These open files are distracting, and people will do what they can to close them. They may call someone else they know, forget all about it, go on vacation, or prescribe medication instead. And if you are hard to get hold of, they will remember that fact next time and be less likely to try your number.

So check your voice mail at least twice a day, and call potential referrals back as soon as you get the message. Suppliers can wait. Colleagues wanting to chat can wait. Committees can wait. But referrals reach their "Best before" date before the sun sets. Make the call.

CORRESPOND WITH REFERRAL SOURCES

Once you have identified your most important referral sources, it's useful to help them keep you in mind for future referrals. There are several ways to do this, mostly involving correspondence with them.

- *Referral thank-you notes:* When you receive a direct referral from another professional, you can write to let the person know that you received the referral, contacted the client, and made an appointment. If (and only if) you have a release signed by the client allowing you to discuss the case with your referral source, you can also let the referring professional know about the outcome of the assessment and the treatment plan. You may or may not routinely send an assessment report. If you don't, a few lines at the bottom of the standard thank-you note may be appreciated and helpful. Enclose a copy of your referral form, your business card, a pamphlet, or all of these.

- *Seasonal cards:* Fewer and fewer people send Christmas cards, but the custom continues in the business world. The holiday season affords a friendly excuse to send a card or note wishing your colleagues well for the new year. In these nonsectarian times, a faith-neutral card is generally best. A brief note is appropriate to include, but generally you would not enclose referral forms or pamphlets with the card.

- *Practice updates:* Changes in your service provide good pretexts for sending notices to your favorite referral sources. Examples include the addition of a new colleague to your practice, changes of address or e-mail contact information, the start-up of a new therapy group, changes in the population you see, new billing procedures, the launch of a new website, and so on. With these announcements, it is entirely appropriate to enclose a pamphlet, card, referral form, or all three.

PRIORITIZE YOUR REFERRAL SOURCES

Not all referral sources are created equal. Some people refer clients to you once a month, others once a year. Some have never referred before, but they represent a strong potential source of future referrals if they like your work. Perhaps you are attempting to cultivate a new line of business, such as rehabilitation work referred by a particular insurance company. Or perhaps there is a certain type of client you love to see, and they tend to be referred to you by a particular agency.

This makes no difference most of the time. You treat everyone well, thank your sources, and deal with people promptly. But sooner or later your service will fill, and you will have to start a waiting list.

It is perfectly legitimate to give different priority to different referral sources. You can leave your referral list open to the sources you like, and close it to others. No need to be deceptive about this: "I'm afraid my service is full at the moment, so I'm accepting referrals only from the transplant clinic in order to prevent people from having to wait too long." You can also be straightforward with the sources you are cultivating: "I really enjoy seeing these clients, so when you refer, we will be making your patients a priority. If our clinical load is full, we'll try to stretch a bit to accommodate them as quickly as possible."

What many do, but you should avoid, is to provide poor service to unloved referral sources—failing to call them back, neglecting to confirm that you have seen referred clients, or adopting a chilly manner on the phone—hoping they will simply go away. This is a needlessly passive-aggressive strategy that should be beneath any responsible practitioner.

Managing a full practice in an active way is not just your right; it is a personal duty. If you sense that you are entirely at the mercy of referral sources—having to accept every client, having to tolerate unprofessional behavior on the part of others, having to take even more of a certain type of client that is driving you toward burnout—then you will not be in practice for long. If the goal is to provide an effective service to as many people as possible, you cannot treat yourself like a therapy machine. Prioritizing is one way to give yourself a sense of personal mastery over your work.

Follow these tips and you will responsibly, ethically, effectively, and appropriately cultivate a referral network. It would be nice if you didn't really have to do any of this, if you could sit behind closed doors, knowing that the knock will come. But it won't. People will come to see you only if they know you exist.

Socially phobic individuals notice that they are friendless and conclude that they are unlovable, so they avoid making social overtures. Clinicians can fall prey to a similar idea: *I'm not getting referrals, so I must be a bad therapist.* Well, you might be; the world is full of incompetent therapists. But it's also possible that you are relying on your expertise and effectiveness to be transmitted telepathically into the minds of prospective clients and referral sources. This is a delusional idea you need to confront and firmly discard.

CHAPTER 5

Creating a Website

Early in the last century, a telephone was an optional extra that a business might have if the owners were what we now call "early adopters." Within a few years, however, a telephone became essential equipment without which doing business was considerably more difficult. Much later, fax machines followed the same trajectory.

Websites have now made the same transition. A website is no longer an option; it is a standard business tool, not unlike a telephone. A business without a website can be an object of suspicion. Is it really a reputable firm? Does it still exist, or has it gone out of business? Just how small is it, anyway?

Professional practices—counselors, accountants, dentists—once lagged behind the rest of the business world in this respect, but they have now caught up. There is no longer a question. You need a website.

This is not a text on Web design, so I will not attempt to cover everything you need to know to develop a website. Instead, this chapter will focus on a few main points, many of them suggested by common mistakes found on psychology and counseling clinic websites. First, though, here are eight reasons to have a site, in case you are not yet convinced:

- When clients are given several clinicians' names, many will look at the providers' websites to learn more and make a selection. If you cannot be found, they will most likely choose one of the names that *can*.

- People increasingly assume that a business has a Web presence, so they may not bother to write down telephone numbers or contact information: "I'll get it off the Web."

- People want to know that they are dealing with a professional who takes their work seriously, and having a website is often seen as an indicator of this.

- Many people get health information from the Internet. If they can glean valuable information from your site, they will tend to see you as an authority.

- An increasing number of people look for a clinician entirely by searching the Internet. At my clinic 40 percent or more of our referrals result from clients looking at our website (without having been referred by anyone else).

- A website is the cheapest form of advertising you will ever purchase. Where else can you make a limitless amount of content accessible to the entire world?

- Any other advertising you do—practice announcements, newspaper ads, your business card, your letterhead—can direct people to your website for more information.

- Ongoing clients will routinely lose your reminder cards and will need to call to verify their appointment times. They'll look for your contact information on your website.

Now, you're a clinician, not a Web designer. If you don't already have a website, the thought of developing one is probably daunting. It needn't be. Let's consider the basics.

DECIDE ON YOUR ADDRESS

Search engines look at all of the content on your site, not just the name. If potential clients don't remember your actual site address, they can still track you down, but you want to make it as easy as possible for people to visit your site and pass the address along to others, so:

Make it short. An address like www.westsidecognitivebehaviourtherapycentre.com is simply too long. The more words, the easier it is to forget one or misspell the name. Also, people checking several options will tend to put off the longest and most complicated address for last. Use as few words as possible.

Make it easy to spell. If your name suggests the website www.laurettapapageorgios.com, try again. No one will remember the spelling.

Avoid words with spelling variants. Examples include "behavior" versus "behaviour," and "counseling" versus "counselling." Your search engine will suggest alternates in search results ("Did you mean *behaviour*?"), but this imposes an additional step in the process of getting to your site.

Avoid acronyms. If your clinic name is a bit long (Portland Stress, Depression, and Wellness Center), you might be tempted to use the initials, but this creates an address that's hard to remember (www.psdwc.com). Drop some words instead: www.portlandstress.com would be much better.

It takes ingenuity to come up with a good website name. Spend some time brainstorming possibilities with family or friends. Write down all of their suggestions and let them percolate in the back of your head for a few days. One morning you will wake up and know what the name should be.

BUY YOUR ADDRESS IMMEDIATELY

Once you have a name, contact your Internet service provider and purchase the address. Do not wait for the website design. You never know when someone else will want that name. "Oh, but it's going to be my name, not something like www.psychology.org." Remember, you are not the only Priscilla Fong in the world. Almost any website name you can think of may be taken at any time.

Which suffix do you want? There are lots to choose from. Here are some observations:

- *.com:* This stands for commercial, and your private practice is a commercial enterprise. This is an entirely appropriate suffix for you. If potential clients remember the name but forget the suffix, this is the first one they'll try.

- *.org:* Generally used for nonprofit and noncommercial sites, this is somewhat less appropriate for a private practice.

- *.info:* This implies that the site is simply an information source, rather than a business. Avoid.

- *.net:* A generic name that is usually used if .com and .org are already taken, but if this is the case, consider switching the name to one for which .com is available.

- *.ca, .au, .uk:* These suffixes indicate the country (other than the United States) where the company is located. Appropriate for a private practice, they are a reasonable alternative to .com. If you get the .com suffix and are located outside the United States, consider purchasing your country's suffix as well, so no one takes it. Some countries offer additional suffixes indicating the organization's state or province: .bc.ca, .on.ca, and so on. This is a needless complication to your website name and takes longer to type. Avoid it.

GENERATE IDEAS FOR CONTENT

What do you put on a website? Take a sheet of paper and visit a colleague's site. List each type of information offered (name, address, and so on). Then visit another site and put check marks beside any type of information from the last site that is on this one as well. At the bottom of the list, add any new content the last site didn't have. Doing this for ten sites will tell you the standard material your colleagues have used and how frequently each part appears. If an item has five check marks beside it, that means it appeared on six of the ten sites, or 60 percent.

Here's some of the information you will find that you might consider for your own site:

- The full name of the practice

- Contact information in all modalities: street address, post-office box address (if applicable), telephone number, fax number, and e-mail address

- Directions to the office, possibly including a map and transit and parking advice

- A picture of the office building, so clients will know it when they see it

- A listing of staff and their clinical specialties, perhaps with photographs of each

- An abbreviated curriculum vitae, or résumé, for each clinician (if you opt to include this, don't post the whole thing)

- Languages in which services are offered

- Wheelchair accessibility

- Significant professional awards received

- Pages on each of the primary activities of the practice: clinical services, workshops, public education events, consulting, or other lines of business

- Difficulties seen, emphasizing your primary specialties

- Background information on the nature of such difficulties

- Whether you handle assessment-only cases, assessment and treatment, or both

- The type of treatment offered and perhaps the treatment philosophy

- Information about payments, including whether you accept credit and debit cards, and how third-party payments are arranged

- An indicator of whether you are currently accepting new clients or have a waiting list

- A statement about whether you require physician referral or accept self-referrals

- A PDF copy of your referral form

- Books you have published, with excerpts if they are written for the general public

- Ordering information for books or other products

- Mass media work you have done, such as interviews or magazine articles

- Upcoming appearances and talks, including talks that are closed to the public or held far away

- Links to other services and relevant organizations

Only a few items on this list are essential, so don't worry if some of them don't fit your practice, or if you want to get started without having to work too hard to develop the site.

What *shouldn't* you include?

- Testimonials from past clients, which are in poor taste and forbidden by many professional organizations (particularly those for psychologists)

- Information that is too breezy or personal; you are a professional and want to communicate this clearly

- Information about unrelated businesses (yes, your spouse may do home renovation work, but this is not the place to advertise it)

THE HOME PAGE

Your home page is the page we see when we type in your Web address (for example, www.madonna.com), which means your home page is the only page that everyone who visits your site will see. On this page, place the content you want every viewer to see.

It's tempting to try to fit all of your content on the home page. All those bits are like your children: it's hard to decide which of them is really important. But your home page is like a lifeboat: you can only fit so much onto it; if you try to stuff everything on it, it will sink. An overly busy home page is overwhelming and confusing to users and will turn them off. So you have to strike a balance between including content and holding it back.

Is it really possible to create a nice, clear home page? Think of the most complicated website there is, the one from which you can access everything on the Net: www.google.com. Most of the home page is blank space. It seems inviting and elegant, not confusing. You may never achieve such elegance, but if a search engine can simplify the entire Web to this extent, surely you can manage with a little private-practice site.

There is another challenge. Every visitor sees only a portion of your home page: the part above the fold. The fold is a reference to newspapers that are folded down the middle. If you are a newspaper editor composing the front page, you put the really important items on the top half of the page so they'll be visible at the kiosk. Slightly less important stories go below the fold on the front page. On a website the part "above the fold" is the content you see in your browser window when you first arrive at a page, without having to scroll down. You have to be extremely careful how you use this one screen. If you try to cram too much onto it, you'll blunt the impact.

When you write content for your home page, you will need to get rid of your usual introductory blather. Look at other clinicians' websites and you'll see how many of them begin with their ideas about life, counseling, mental illness, or their dog Mr. Pickles: "Welcome to Sunrise Counseling. We believe that life can be a difficult endeavor for any of us, and…" You can stop there, because the viewer has already clicked over to someone else's site.

Take the viewpoint of the potential client visiting your site. Why are you there? What do you really want? Give it to your viewers quickly or show immediately where they can get it. When I first designed my own website, I was tempted to review the history of the clinic. Eventually I realized my mistake and shifted this content to another page, replacing it with "Welcome to Changeways Clinic. We offer three things: therapy services, products, and training workshops." Each of those three things was a link to a separate section of the site.

PREPARE FOR THE DESIGN

Make a list of everything you want to include on your website, perhaps placing each item on a separate index card. Do not worry about the order, placement, or relative importance of the material at this stage. As the deck of cards gets thicker, you may experience some anxiety at the magnitude of the task before you. Relax. Remind yourself that you need not do it all at once. Your website is like an infinitely expandable parking garage. Your task is simply to outline the entryway and the first floor. More floors can be added later. The bits of content are like the cars in the garage: they can be added as you go, and the structure does not depend on them.

You may notice a fear that you will overdo the content in some areas and neglect others, producing an inelegant and lopsided result. This is a problem in an essay but not in a website. No one sees the full structure, so if you include much more on one topic than another, most people will never notice.

Once you have generated your stack of index cards, lay them out on a large table. Select the cards representing material that should appear on your home page. Put all of these at the far-left side of the table. It's all right if you are a bit overinclusive, but you will soon have to cut it back.

Next, look at what remains. Group the cards together by theme. These themes will create the major sections of your site. Some themes might be "The Problems We Treat," "About Cognitive Therapy," "Presentations and Workshops," "About Us," and "Consulting Services for Organizations." Try to get everything into two to eight main themes where possible. More than this will probably be confusing for site users.

Some themes, such as "About Cognitive Therapy," might be presented on a single page. Other themes will incorporate a great deal of material and will best be presented across multiple pages. For example, perhaps your "Presentations and Workshops" theme will branch into "For Professionals" and "For the General Public," with several programs in each category, and your "About Us" theme will have separate pages with your staff list, your contact information, and any history or background on your service that you want to include. Perhaps a few of your themes will have sub-subthemes. Unless your site is very elaborate, however, you don't want more than about four levels (home page, theme pages, subthemes, sub-subthemes).

Your groups of cards may have made a few new pages necessary. You've put together all of the cards describing the various anxiety disorders, for example, so now you need a page called something like "About Anxiety," from which they can branch.

Once you have found places for all of your cards, write the design on paper. Use one line per page, and indicate the level of each page with setbacks. Following is an example of a clinic offering therapy, continuing education for professionals, and talks for the general public. No page is more than three clicks from the home page. By using pull-down menus, you could reduce this to two clicks, or even one.

Home Page	Major Theme	Subtheme	Sub-Subtheme
Home			
	For Clients		
		Difficulties Seen	
			About Depression
			About Bulimia
			About Anorexia
		About Cognitive Therapy	
		Setting Appointments	
		Financial Details	
	For Professionals		
		How to Refer	

			Referral Form (PDF)	
			About Workshops	
				Workshops Offered
				How to Host a Program
		Calendar		
			Upcoming Public Talks	
			Upcoming Professional Talks	
			Past Presentations	
		About Us		
			Staff	
			Our History	
			Contact Information	
		Links		

Next, put a star beside the pages that you absolutely need to have on the site before you launch it. It's fine if some pages read "Under Construction" for a while. Your primary agenda is to get a Web presence; you can fine-tune it later.

Start writing the text for the pages you really need. Again, you will be tempted to use your normal writing style: introduction, content, conclusion. Try to set this aside and simply write the content itself. If it's confusing or needs background, you can insert a link users can click to learn more. In the course of writing, you may discover a few more pages you need or will eventually want.

AVOID ANIMATION AND WELCOME SCREENS

People who are new to website design often become fascinated with the process and want to add lots of artwork and animation. They often like the idea of a "front door" that displays something inviting to the viewer before shifting to the more functional home page.

Avoid such temptations. No one will visit your site to see your art, your animations, or your flowing graphics or inspirational quotes. Forcing them to sit through your welcome screen is a self-indulgent act of disrespect to the very people you hope to serve. It's like the hidden message of telemarketers: "Your time is so unimportant that we think you have nothing better to do than listen to our advertising."

People go to websites to get information, so give it to them. Take a look at some of the most successful websites, such as www.amazon.com and www.wikipedia.org: no animation, no welcome-to-our-site slide show. If you want artwork on your site, fine; put it off to one side of the real content, or provide a link to it. But don't irritate your site visitors as the first thing you do. No one will be more likely to use your service because you showed a picture of your cat first.

HIRE A DESIGNER

You may think this suggestion should have appeared earlier in this chapter. Wrong. A Web designer cannot tell you what services you offer, who your clients are, or what they want to learn from your site. All of that is up to you. Once you have identified the major sections of your site and come up with some of your content, however, it's time to bring in someone to help.

Why get help? Because you are in business to practice, not to fuss with website design. If you try to create your own site, you will spend days trying to figure things out, and you'll wind up with something that looks distressingly homemade. For less time and money (if you consider what your time is actually worth), you can get something better.

Whom should you hire? This is one instance where the old saying "You get what you pay for" isn't true. The more money you spend, the less likely you will get what you need. Choose someone with a good understanding of the basics, and avoid professionals who want to dazzle you with their creativity. Your clients don't want to admire your page design. They want to know what street you're on. Be explicit that you want an inexpensive, fast-loading, no-nonsense website.

One thing you *do* want is the ability to add pages and change content yourself. You shouldn't have to call your designer every time you add a new colleague or schedule a public talk. If there is a conflict between anyone's vision and the user-friendliness of updating the content, updating takes clear priority.

Note that if you are going to have high-security content on the website, you want higher-end help. For example, if you want a site where people type in their credit card information to buy things, you will want to ensure that it is properly designed. Very few mental health practitioners have sites like this, however.

MAKE IT SIMPLE TO NAVIGATE

A lot of websites have wonderful content that few people ever see because the sites are so difficult to navigate. Users either look at a few pages, unaware that much more is available, or curse the designer while trying to find their way around.

How do you make a website more navigable? Use standard buttons and menus. Creative menu design is unhelpful, because users click around the page trying to find what they need.

Also, branches from one topic area to the next should generally not have too many options. A page-long option list tends to be overwhelming. If you limit yourself to six subtheme options from any page and four levels (as in the example earlier in the chapter), you can have 259 pages (including the home page). That's far more than any clinician is ever likely to need.

How can you verify that your site is easy to navigate? Recruit a not-so-Web-savvy friend and have the person try to find his way around. Set your friend specific tasks, like "Find my picture," "What's the date of my next talk?" and "Imagine that you're a physician who wants the referral form." Watch what your friend does. Don't help. Look for hesitation, wrong moves, and confusion. Rather than attribute the issue to your friend's lousy problem-solving skills, recognize that your site is the problem. Fix it. Remember that prospective clients may visit the site in a state of agitation and distress. Could they still find their way around?

TEST IT ON ALL WEB BROWSERS

So you design your site and create a mock-up, and it looks great. Unfortunately, the site may look different on different browsers. Upload the site to the Web and navigate to it using every browser you can. Ensure that you try a PC, a Mac, and a smartphone, and that you look around and try all the buttons. Feel proud of yourself for doing this. A certain national airline with a maple leaf on the tail found it to be beyond their abilities.

If there is a problem, it will be a mission for your designer, because it will likely prove to be beyond your own skills. Note that the more complicated your site design, the more likely you are to have browser issues. This is yet another reason to go for a very simple design.

DO NOT HAVE A BLOG

A Weblog, or blog, can be a fun thing to read and can encourage viewers to return to a website again and again. Many therapists are frustrated authors, so a blog can be tempting. After all, it's standard advice to update your website content regularly. We've all seen those sites that obviously haven't been tended in ages, announcing talks "Upcoming in 2006." It is a good idea to tend your site regularly and keep it reasonably up to date.

But why do you have a website? You are not really trying to maximize hits. Your site is designed to inform people about your services and tell them how to get in contact with you, and that's about it. Spending a lot of time fussing over your return readership is a distraction from your business, not an addition to it.

That said, having a good website may make it more likely that someone will schedule an appointment with you, hire you as a consultant or public speaker, or look you up for a media interview. Short articles presenting your perspective on key issues related to your practice can be interesting and helpful: "Do Antidepressants Work?" "Exercise and Mood," "Recent Findings About Panic." Feel free to post them, but don't call your posts a blog. This way you have something extra to offer your site visitors, but without the guilt.

Having a blog turns this option into an obligation. You will feel pressure to write regularly, and the time will become steadily harder to find. Rather than feel the liberation of having a creative outlet, you will have created yet another stick for your superego to beat you with. You have a busy life. If you don't, then the point of the website is to make it busier by inviting more people to purchase your services, not by occupying you with non–revenue-producing time wasters.

THE LINKS PAGE

One way to increase your page's profile is to have it link to a number of other sites. What should you link to, though? Your practice's website is not a personal site, so select links that actually relate to your business. Here are some options:

- *Mental health information sites:* Include sites that provide reputable information on the main difficulties you see or the therapeutic modalities you practice.

- *Professional organizations:* Consider providing links to your local professional practice organization, the national organization, and others. Many of these sites include referral services and information sheets on diverse issues.

- *Consumer advocacy and education organizations:* Consumer-run organizations are available for people facing many concerns. They often provide a useful perspective that complements professional information sources.

- *Lifestyle resources:* If you frequently recommend that people try out certain activities, you could provide links to the related websites. Examples include your local tourism information site, the night-school section of the local school-board site, and the area's community center listings.

- *Local mental health or social service information:* Many clients need additional services, such as addiction treatment centers or women's shelters. You can provide links to these services or to your region's service directory on your site.

This is just a sampling of the possibilities. There are many more. When you add a local organization to your site, drop them a line and let them know. They may wish to link to your site in return. Include a standard paste-in paragraph describing your site, so they don't have to visit it to make a decision whether to link to you. Also consider having links open in a new browser window rather than take your viewer away from your own site.

MAXIMIZE HITS

The whole point of having a website is to get visitors to read it and possibly purchase your service. Some people will have your Web

Creating a Website

address and type it straight into their browser. A larger number will find your site using a search engine. Consequently, it is important for your site to come up high in the list of search results.

Your ranking in search results depends partly on the frequency with which people visit your site (a catch-22 type of problem), partly on the words visibly appearing within your site, and (for some browsers) partly on the keywords you add to the site. Your designer will know how to put keywords into your site but won't know what terms people are most likely to use when searching for your site. That part is up to you. Avoid adding keywords that do not actually appear on a given page, because this may cause the page to be rejected by the search engine. The best words depend on the type of service you provide, but here are some suggestions:

- Your name, including the most common misspellings you've noticed

- Your location, by town, region, and province or state (Moncton, Okanagan, Illinois)

- Your profession (counselor, psychologist, social worker)

- Your service (therapy, psychotherapy, counseling)

- The type of therapy or service you provide (cognitive, behavioral)

- The population you see (children, seniors, obsessive-compulsive disorder, OCD, autism, autistic, Asperger's).

Once you have launched your site, use several search engines to try to find it. Imagine that you are a client who has only a vague notion of the spelling of your name and the service sought. Get your friends to try to find your site, but don't tell them more about your work than your prospective clients or referral sources would know. If you don't appear routinely on the first page of search results, go back to the drawing board and consult with your designer.

MAKE YOUR CONTACT INFO EASY TO ACCESS

Obviously your contact information should be a part of your website. But where should you put it? Answer: your contact information is the most important thing on the site. It should be everywhere.

Too many clinicians' websites hide the contact information as though it were an Easter egg they didn't want to be found. Don't make the rookie mistake of placing your contact info only on a subpage ("How to Contact Us") within another section ("About Us"). This may seem perfectly understandable to you, but it takes the viewer a moment or two to think of it. Instead, make your contact information a part of *every* page. One option is to put it just beneath your menu or on a sidebar, plainly visible "above the fold" in a section that appears on every page. Alternatively, add it in a smaller font at the bottom of every page, where many Web pages have a subsidiary list of links.

※

This is only a short list of the considerations involved in creating your website. Your designer can provide you with more. Do not feel intimidated, however. Websites are not difficult to design, and most of the major pitfalls are fairly easy to avoid. Make it simple, make it easy, and don't let your Web designer get too fancy on you.

Remember that a website is utterly unlike most other projects you have ever attempted. You would never write a few paragraphs and then send an incomplete article off to a journal. You would never move into a home before the plumbing was in. But a website becomes functional with a minimum of content. You can upload it to the Web with only a page or two of material and then add more at your leisure. Run your ideas past a few colleagues and the all-important teenage technophiles. Then get your foothold in the twenty-first century.

CHAPTER 6

Managing Client Information

For almost ten years I supervised students in a predoctoral internship program. Occasionally interns would express frustration about some of the mechanical aspects of their work. They couldn't find file folders. They couldn't get hold of clients who had been referred. The referring physician wouldn't call them back. They spent an inordinate amount of time trying to keep their files straight. This wasn't how they wanted to spend their time. They were there to learn assessment and therapy. Everything else was a distraction. During their earlier practicum work, they had simply shown up, met with the supervisor, and toddled in to see clients, whose appointments had been set up for them in advance.

The truth is that in practicum settings, supervisors were willing to trust students to provide clinical services, provided they had the usual supervision. But students were not trusted with the management of client flow and information. At the internship program we did not have the administrative staff to do everything for them, and we wanted them to learn to manage files properly.

This chapter is concerned with the issue of managing clients apart from delivering clinical services. In many years of school, I heard not a peep on this topic (apart from a few words about release of information forms). But as essential as what you do when clients are in the room is what you do before and after they are there.

ASSIGN A NUMBER TO EACH CLIENT

Our clients are human beings: complex, multifaceted, unique entities that cannot be reduced to numbers or *DSM-IV* diagnostic codes. We avoid referring to them as "My OCD at three o'clock." So assigning them numbers seems cold, inappropriate, and contradictory. Why do it?

Material related to clients appears in computer records, letters, test documents, supervision tapes, and financial spreadsheets and on insurance billing forms. All of these documents must be kept secure, but each represents an opportunity for the client's private information to be spread inadvertently. For the sake of confidentiality, it is good practice to minimize the number of places where clients' names appear. The best way to do this is to assign a number to each client.

At my own clinic we assign each client a number that begins with the year in which we first see the person (say, 2011). Following a dash, a number is assigned, representing the order in which that client was seen that year, and then the client's initials appear. This would give the first new client of 2011, Harpo Marx, the number 2011-001HM.

Problem: clients often see their numbers, and at first my private practice was a part-time affair. "Hang on, I started seeing you in February, and my number is 1998-002DC. Did you only see two people that year?" I got around this by starting with the number 100. So the first person for 2011 is really 2011-101HM. Harpo keeps this number for as long as he comes to the clinic.

The client number is used as much as possible in place of the client's name. The file folder is labeled with the number and the client's first name and last initial. Computer files with client information are named using the client number as well. Here are some examples:

2011-101HMan: The initial assessment note

2011-101HMn: Ongoing session notes

2011-101HMbill: Client bills and receipts

2011-101HMgoals: Weekly goal-setting records

2011-101HMhier: Exposure hierarchy for Harpo's phobia treatment

2011-101HMtn: Termination note from the conclusion of therapy

USE A DEMOGRAPHIC INFORMATION FORM

There is absolutely no point in wasting most of a client's first session taking down information the client can write at home or in the waiting room ahead of time. Consequently, it's a good idea to create and use a simple demographic information form.

What should the form ask for? Some suggestions follow (a sample of a "Confidential Client Information" form is available at the websites noted in the introduction). Content in parentheses could appear on the form itself; content in square brackets is my commentary. Some of the later items are specific to therapy practices; coaches and those offering other services may wish to substitute content of their own.

- *Your* [that is, the client's] *complete name.*

- *Address.*

- *Home phone and daytime contact numbers (please circle any number where we can leave a message).*

- *E-mail address (optional).*

- *Birth date [you will need the birth date to identify the client for most billing and for identifying the client to a referring physician].*

- *Birthplace [this signals the client's immigration history, which can often be a significant factor in therapy].*

- *Education (grade completed, plus any postsecondary education).*

- *Gender [leave a blank line rather than "M/F," so transgendered clients can take the opportunity to let you know here].*

- *Occupation.*

- *Person to alert in the event of medical emergency, their relationship to you, and their phone number [you will almost never need this, but you must have it on file].*

- *Family physician and phone number.*

- *Relationship status (circle): single, married, partnered, separated, divorced, widowed ["partnered" is included for common-law couples and in regions not yet permitting same-sex marriage].*

- *Partner's first name, age, years in relationship.*

- *Children (please note gender and age).*

- *Please describe any significant current or past medical problems.*

- *Please list any medications you currently take, including prescription and over-the-counter medications and the dosage of each [allow at least four lines for this].*

Managing Client Information

- *Have you had previous psychological care or counseling?*

- *If yes, please give the name of the clinician(s), when you were seen (for example, Nov. '06–Feb. '08), and the nature of the difficulty at the time* [leave at least four lines].

- *Have you ever been hospitalized for a psychological difficulty?*

- *If yes, please give the dates and the nature of the difficulty at the time.*

- *In your own words, what is the nature of the concern that you wish to address in therapy? Feel free to describe this in as much or as little detail as you wish. Use additional paper if you like.* [Allow at least six lines. Replies to this item will tell you a lot.]

- *Therapy can be a powerful force for change. In order for therapy to be most effective, it helps to have a clear and specific goal. You may find it difficult to express your hopes for therapy in the form of a goal, but please make at least an initial effort. You can discuss this further with your therapist. Feel free to list more than one goal if you wish.* [Allow at least six lines. This question communicates that the client is an active participant and needs to be thinking about the direction of therapy.]

A form with all of these questions will run to three pages. People sometimes ask if this isn't asking too much of a client at the outset. At our clinic we have never had a client object to the form, and clients seldom fail to complete it before the first session. If we mail it to them ahead of time and they forget to bring it, we ask them to complete a new copy in the waiting room when they arrive. Don't ask them to bring it next time. If clients forget to bring something to the first appointment, it is unlikely they will bring it to the second.

It is vital to let clients know that their own input is the active ingredient in therapy. If the client can't take a primary role, therapy will not work. The best way to communicate this is verbally (in the first session) *and* nonverbally via the implicit assumption that clients will be willing to do a bit of work at the outset.

Of course, if you suspect that the client has literacy problems, ask gently before mailing the form: "Would you be able to complete that for our next meeting?" "Some people have difficulties with reading or eyesight; is that a concern?" For clients who are concerned about confidentiality, give them the option to "fill in whatever you feel comfortable writing down, and we can discuss anything else when we meet."

GET A SIGNED RELEASE OF INFORMATION FORM

Most physicians don't seem to have a big problem with the release of client information. Specialists routinely send reports back to the referring physician without letting the patient know they are doing so. Other clinicians should be more careful. We must get a signed release of information form that allows us to talk with other professionals.

It's tempting to think that we can tell in advance when we will need one of these forms. If we want to discuss medication with the physician, we can get the form then. If the client is sliding into a paranoid psychotic break or developing an erotomanic obsession with the therapist, we will see it coming. Much of therapy is about identifying persuasive and intuitive but utterly wrong assumptions about the world. This is one of them. I can't tell with any reliability when I will want or need a release, and neither can you.

Having had a few unusual experiences, I now get a release of information form signed for just about every client I see. When I have the sense that "I won't really need this, so why bother?" I ignore it immediately. Find out whether your jurisdiction has a standard legal form you would have to use. If not, create your own and run it past a lawyer. Use it religiously, and introduce it within minutes of first meeting the client. Never run out.

USE A LIMITS TO CONFIDENTIALITY FORM

It's easy to get a broken toe treated without having to worry a great deal about confidentiality. Who cares if the world finds out? When clients see a therapist, however, they will almost certainly discuss information they would not want shared with the world. This may cause them to withhold information. Alternatively, they may assume that anything they say to a therapist is absolutely privileged, and they will be shocked and enraged (and possibly litigious) should this prove incorrect.

Consequently, it's important for a therapist to spell out the limitations of confidentiality with all clients during the first session. These limitations vary by jurisdiction and profession, so please do not assume that the ones mentioned here apply in your case or represent the complete list in your own region. Common limits include:

- If the client is judged to be at serious risk of doing significant self-harm or harm to someone else
- If the client reports information indicating that a child is being or is at risk of being abused
- If the client holds a driver's license and is not fit to operate a motor vehicle
- If the therapist is subpoenaed by a court of law

There are other issues:

- *Age of consent:* If you see children or teenagers, the parents or legal guardian may have access to the client's file. The age at which they have the relatively complete confidentiality of an adult varies by region.
- *Competence:* If you see people who may not be legally competent (such as some individuals with dementia, chronic psychosis, or serious brain injury), their legal guardian might have access to the file.

- *Couples and family therapy:* If you see both members of a couple, your notes will likely include information about both parties, and both will most likely have the legal right of access to the file. The same may be true of families. You would be best advised to spell this out, including your inability to guarantee the confidentiality of anything one party says when the other is out of the room.

How should you create a form that suits your own region, profession, practice, and population? The best course of action is to consult your ethical guidelines to develop an initial sense of what to include. Then discuss the issue with long-established colleagues or those who have recently taken registration examinations (and so might have such knowledge close at hand). Finally, run your tentative form past someone in your profession's governing body or a legal representative of your practice's insurer.

USE A CONSENT TO TREATMENT FORM

Once you have assessed clients and they seem appropriate and amenable to treatment, you will commence with therapy. But the client may not know what therapy entails or may have unrealistic expectations for the outcome. It's important to clarify the client's understanding of the process, some of which will be done verbally, when you review the nature of the client's problem and discuss what you think might be helpful. Some of it, however, should be spelled out in a consent to treatment form that you will ask the client to sign.

What should go in your consent to treatment form? Here are some of the bases to cover:

- The type of treatment you do. A paragraph should suffice.
- A statement about the research supporting or underlying your model.
- A clear statement that no therapy can guarantee results.

- A statement that therapy can stir up powerful emotions in a person and that the goal of therapy is not necessarily to avoid this.

- A statement that simply coming in to talk with the therapist is not sufficient to produce change. Improvement requires that the client make therapy a priority by attending sessions and by selecting and carrying out activities between sessions as well (that is, if your model includes this feature).

- A statement about your no-show policy. Is a missed session billable? Most practitioners bill for sessions not canceled at least twenty-four hours in advance.

- A statement about payments. Is the client expected to pay at each session, once a month, or by some other arrangement? If the client fails to pay within a specified period of time, is interest charged? Can the bill be turned over to a collection agency?

- You can incorporate the list of limitations to confidentiality and the consent to release information into your consent to treatment form if you wish, in order to minimize paperwork.

When should you present the consent to treatment form? Common practice in some jurisdictions (check the recommended practice in your own area) is to hold off until the end of the first assessment session. If you do this, be sure to do two things:

- Remind clients that the assessment phase involves a lot of questions, and they should feel free to decline to answer any questions they wish.

- If the limitations to confidentiality are incorporated into the consent to treatment form, review them verbally at the beginning of the first meeting, and make a note that you have done so.

WHAT TO PUT IN A FIRST SESSION NOTE

Most clinicians go through extensive training programs in which they are required to write lengthy assessment notes. If you conduct assessments for third-party insurers, or if the assessment is the primary service being offered, you may well want to produce an extensive assessment note. For most therapy clients, however, the referral source seldom expects a detailed note. At most, they want to know your basic findings and what you plan to do.

That said, professionals must keep adequate notes on their work, and you will want an account of the assessment to which you can refer back and from which you can generate a longer note if required. If you aren't going to write a five-page report, what should you do?

Most professional organizations require that certain information be on file. Some of this, such as an emergency contact number and the client's full name and date of birth, are listed on the demographic information form, and there is no need to repeat it.

It's a good idea to have a blank "Assessment Note" file that you can open and tailor for each new client by simply filling in the blanks. Here are some possible headings:

- Client number and name.

- Date of initial assessment.

- Referral source.

- Current situation, including the client's age, home situation, employment, relationship status, and other pertinent information about the present state of affairs.

- Nature and history of presenting problem. If there is more than one problem, use a paragraph to describe each. Note current symptoms and characteristics, the developmental history of the problem, and pertinent risk factors thus far identified.

- Presentation. Note characteristics, including manner of dress, promptness or lateness, anomalies of movement, facial expression, lability of mood in session, response to questioning, ability as a personal historian, mental status, self-care and hygiene, orientation to treatment (*Does he seem eager to get help? Does she expect the therapist to take over and solve the problem? Is he here by his own choice?*), and apparent psychological state (for example, suspicion, discouragement, cheerfulness).

- Test results. Any scores or interpretation of psychometric tests or behavioral monitoring.

- Other conditions, substances, lifestyle factors. Note any physical illnesses or other difficulties not previously mentioned (such as diabetes, obesity, mild flight phobia). Substance use (including alcohol, nicotine, and caffeine) is recorded. Lifestyle factors are touched on briefly, including exercise regimen, sleep hygiene, diet, social life and support, incorporation of enjoyable activity into daily life, and work style (such as a tendency to overwork).

- Treatment history. Focus on psychological and psychiatric interventions for the current or any previous disorder, including hospitalization and medications, with a careful inventory of all medications currently being taken.

- Plan. Note initial impressions and a rough outline of the interventions thought likely to be of use. The plan is unlikely to be complete after a single assessment session, but it should provide guidance for the first few steps.

One item seems to be missing from this list: the formulation. You can write any provisional ideas you have at the start of the "Plan" section, but you are unlikely to have a complete formulation after a single assessment session. The note is designed to remind you of the salient points you will want to take into account after the second or third session. The lack of a precise formulation does not prevent you from coming up with a tentative plan for the very early stage of therapy. It doesn't take a great deal of insight to know that becoming more active and getting out of the house now and then will be a good idea for a depressed individual, or that some sort of exposure-based work is likely to be part of the plan for a person with an anxiety disorder. A more complete formulation should appear as part of the note for the second or third session.

ONGOING SESSION NOTES

Once you shift from assessment to treatment, note taking becomes somewhat easier. My own session notes are usually a quarter to a third of a typed, single-spaced page. What should you include?

- Date.
- If the client was late and, if so, by how many minutes.
- The client's emotional state at the outset of the appointment, either by observation or by the client's own report.
- A review of goal setting or other therapeutic work since the last appointment.
- Significant events since the last appointment.
- Therapeutic tasks completed in session.
- Any significant reactions or insights in session.
- Homework set by the client or suggested by the clinician.
- Plan for the next appointment.
- Whether or not the client has paid.
- Clinician's signature. If you are in a solo practice, your governing organization may or may not require this for

each note, because it is clear that everyone is seen by you. In a multiple-provider clinic, a signature is advisable.

HANDLING REQUESTS FOR INFORMATION

You may never be called on to attend court and, if you are, you will want more guidance than this book provides. There is no escaping the fact, however, that sooner or later, lawyers or third-party insurers will ask you for your clinical records.

An in-depth examination of the issue is beyond the scope of this book, but the matter is discussed in Gerald Koocher and Patricia Keith-Spiegel's book *Ethics in Psychology and the Mental Health Professions* (2008) and in an article by the American Psychological Association's Committee on Legal Issues (2006). One basic principle, however, is to provide the least amount of information possible, at least to the initial request.

Lawyers almost always request a photocopy of the entire client file: session notes, billing information, questionnaire data, and all. Perhaps they do this because, every now and then, a practitioner immediately gives them everything. Any ethical wrongdoing will be the fault of the practitioner, not the lawyer who asked.

The first thing to do is to check to see if your client provided you a release of information form. A letter from a lawyer is not the same as a subpoena, so it does not override your client's confidentiality rights. Feel free to reject a form that you can't read, that does not identify you or your clinic as a source of information, or that includes nothing but a chicken scratch that may or may not be your client's signature.

Next, call the client yourself to verify that she knows the request has been made. Clients are often surprised that the therapist has been asked for information, and you can tell them that you will provide nothing without their explicit permission (or a subpoena). Consider asking the client whether she would be willing to complete your own release of information form, identifying the lawyer who is making the request. If you are not satisfied with the permission form the lawyer supplied, you cannot fall back on the client's verbal agreement over the telephone.

Sometimes clients will be in a rush, either because events have happened precipitously or because they have procrastinated over the legal process and are now working against a tight deadline. Never use this as a reason to skip getting a form signed and in hand before giving out information.

What should you do once you have a release in hand? Read the actual request carefully, ensuring that you do not provide any information beyond what was explicitly requested. My colleague William Koch (2009) advises:

> *Don't be afraid to call up the requester and seek clarification (obviously with the consent of your client); for example, "What do you want from the file?" The requester—the lawyer or insurer, for example—may be quite frank and say something like, "We need to know what they were being treated for," or alternatively, "We need access to psychological test data for our independent consultant to review." This brings some clarity to those threatening blanket releases and may suggest ways to satisfy the request without unduly exposing your client to prejudicial information being released.*

Beyond this, practitioners vary in their approach, and the best strategy is to consult established professionals in your jurisdiction and field. My own policy is to give as little information as possible. If this is not satisfactory, whoever's seeking the information can always write back for more. I very seldom get a follow-up letter.

What I write varies depending on what was requested. The most common request is for the complete file and all session notes. I never provide them in response to an initial request and have never been pursued for them (though I do not make a practice of taking medicolegal cases). Instead, I write a note listing the dates on which the client was seen and a brief sketch of the service provided. If there was

Managing Client Information

a diagnosis involved, I may provide it. I offer no speculation in this type of document and do not elaborate on the basics. I am not being paid for a consultation note, so I do not write one.

Lawyers' notes almost always offer a fee for your time in preparing the information for them. Charge it. They typically do not quote a dollar figure, so bill your regular hourly rate multiplied by the time spent. If you bill for more than an hour, they may decline to pay, claiming that they did not request a specially written report, just copies of what already existed in the file. As well, if you spend more than an hour writing the note, you are probably providing more information than is necessary. If you do not bill, you show that you will work for the lawyer at no charge, and the person will probably take you up on it again.

Ethics seminars and books are filled with answers to questions about trickier issues: What if a subpoena requests the original copyrighted questionnaire forms? What if the client has you write a report, then provides information contradicting your earlier impression and denies you permission to revise or withdraw your note? What if you are convinced that the information you provide will run counter to the best interests of your client? Find and read a good reference book on the legal issues you will most likely encounter in your own type of practice.

One last caution: you will occasionally get a client who asks you to tamper with his record. Never do this. In most cases this is illegal, and it is certainly unethical. All of the responsibility for these acts lies with the practitioner, not with the person making the request. Although it is entirely appropriate to be circumspect about what you put in the file in the first place, once it is there and has been requested, it is too late to take it out or alter it.

MAKE CLIENT FILES EASILY RECOGNIZABLE

You will have all kinds of files in your office, and you will have busy days when a lot of material winds up on your desk. You can spend an

127

inordinate amount of time looking for things, and you will want to be especially careful with your client files. Consequently, it's a good idea to make different kinds of information easy to spot.

One option is to code different kinds of files with stickers, like the simple colored dots available from any stationery store. The problem is that they are small and don't cause the entire file to pop out at you from across the room. A better solution is to use colored file folders. The system at my clinic reflects the activities we do, so it may not fit your own needs. Nevertheless, here it is:

- Navy blue: Client files

- Light blue: Clinic administration

- Gray: Clinic finances

- Red: Workshop registration files

- Green: Presentations other than revenue-producing workshops

- Purple: Document masters for the print shop

- Orange: Consulting services

- Plain: Everything that does not fit readily into one of the preceding categories, including research materials and journal articles

This list may be overelaborative for those with a less complicated business. The fewer divisions you have, the more likely you will be to keep with the system rather than give up when you run out of folders of a given color.

At minimum, get a contrasting color for client files. It's important that you be able to find them, and at the end of the day, you want to be particularly careful to make sure they are locked away. A quick glance at your desk will tell you whether you have done this.

ORGANIZE THE FILE

Client files start out slim and wind up thick with paper. It's tempting to think, *Looking through a file doesn't take all that long.* But if you measured the bits of time you spend hunting through client files in a year, you would discover that you have lost a day or more. Developing a ritualized scheme for maintaining order in the file is more than worthwhile. It verges on an ethical requirement. Here's one system:

- Identify the file with the client number, first name, and last initial; for example, "2010-147 John S."

- Staple the client's referral form (if any) and demographic information form to the inside left of the folder.

- Attach your session notes atop the demographic form with a grip clip, with the most recent ones topmost (this makes it easier to add new notes).

- Clip test results to the right side of the file.

- Use grip clips to bind thematically related sheets in the file: things like notes from the physician, legal forms, copies of other professionals' reports, behavioral monitoring sheets, goal-setting forms, and so on.

The first two months you do this, you will think you are wasting your time (and lots of grip clips), but from then until the end of your career, you will be glad you made this a habit.

DEVELOP YOUR OWN SHORTHAND

Psychotherapy involves a lot of note taking. Some therapists manage to remember the details of a session until the client leaves the room, never writing anything down. Others make occasional rough notes during a session and then create formal notes afterward, shredding the draft. There are even rumors of a third species: the clinician who can take lovely, coherent notes while the client is in the room. When the client leaves, all this clinician has to do is put the sheet into the client's file.

Regardless of which type you are, you will want to develop your note-taking skills. The faster you can write, the better your in-session notes will be and the less they will distract you from the client. You will also be able to write up more extensive postsession notes before your next client arrives. Using your own standard abbreviations can speed you up, and they eventually become so automatic you don't have to think about them.

Problem: others must be able to read your session notes. Consequently, you should either use your shorthand only for rough notes or, if you use it for your final notes, include a code sheet in each client's file.

If you adopt this idea, you will want to use your own system. You will use terms, clinical instruments, and techniques that others do not. Table 6.1 provides a sample system in which the abbreviations are divided into categories (a copy is available at the websites noted in the introduction). Many of the abbreviations are obvious and common; a few are not.

Table 6.1 A Sample Abbreviation System for Client Notes

PEOPLE		COMMON WORDS	
Capitalized initials. Usually, client's name		appt.	Appointment
		attn.	Attention
+4, -3.	Usually, the age of a person relative to client	avail.	Available
		beh.	Behavior
bf.	Boyfriend	co.	Company
gf.	Girlfriend	conv.	Conversation
bro.	Brother	disc.	Discussion
sis.	Sister	E.	Experiment
sib.	Sibling	emot.	Emotion
ch.	Child	empl.	Employed, employment
ct.	Client	enc.	Encourage, encouraged
f.	Father	ex.	Example
m.	Mother	exer.	Exercise
hus.	Husband	fr.	From, friend (context)
wf.	Wife	frus.	Frustrated, frustration
mgf.	Maternal grandfather	fu.	Follow-up (of previous work)
mgm.	Maternal grandmother		
pgf.	Paternal grandfather	hr.	Hour
pgm.	Paternal grandmother	imm.	Immediate
		incl.	Including
		inted.	Interested
		L.	Language
		max.	Maximum
		min.	Minimum, minute

DOCUMENTS		COMMON WORDS	
24hr diary	Record form requesting activities each hour	neg.	Negative
		pd.	Paid
5col.	Five-column cognitive challenging form	phys.	Physical, physiological
		pos.	Positive
BAI	Beck Anxiety Inventory	re.	About
		reass.	Reassurance
BDI	Beck Depression Inventory II	rec.	Recommend, recommended
PAI	Personality Assessment Inventory	rel.	Relaxation
		reln.	Relationship
THERAPY TASKS AND INTERVENTIONS		RTW	Return to work
		sch.	School
adepr.	Antidepressant	sitn.	Situation
benz.	Benzodiazepine	soc.	Social
cogintro.	Discussion of cognitive therapy concepts	sugg.	Suggest, suggested
		tho.	Though
diabr.	Diaphragmatic breathing training	thot.	Thought
		ult.	Ultimate
emotintro.	Discussion of emotional tolerance concepts	v.	Very
		w.	With
		w/o	Without
ERP	Exposure and response prevention	wk.	Week or work (context)
h/o	Information handout		
med.	Medication		
PMR	Progressive muscle relaxation		
strman.	Stress management concepts		

HAVE ACTIVE AND INACTIVE FILE STORAGE

At first we see clients regularly, so we want their files close at hand. Eventually we stop seeing some clients, and their files become a distraction. Consequently, you will probably want to have a second storage area for inactive files.

Once all outstanding issues (such as receipt of payment or completion of a termination note) are resolved, strip the file of any nonessential material, add the client's full last name to the file label (if it isn't there already), and file it by last name in the "Inactive" file cabinet, which might be in your assistant's office. Should the client call in, the file can be easily found and forwarded to you for action.

It is essential that both active and inactive file areas be secure. It is not sufficient for files to be behind a locked door; cleaning staff have access to every room but should not have access to client information. It is the clinician's responsibility to take all reasonable measures to ensure that client confidentiality is not compromised.

Eventually you may find you have so many inactive files that it is no longer practical to store them on-site. It may become essential to rent a secure storage area with a reputable firm or to contract with a record-storage company. It is up to you to make sure the company has appropriate security measures in place to prevent theft. To make sure you won't often have to hunt through documents stored off-site, you might wish to subdivide your inactive files into two categories: files that may well be reactivated at some point, and files that are almost certain never to be used again. You would then keep the former at your own office, and have a list of all those kept off-site.

If you store inactive files off-site, you may be obliged to inform your professional organization where these documents might be found. Check your organization's guidelines on this point.

CLEAN OUT YOUR OWN FILES

Files can accumulate litter: your chicken-scratch notes, phone messages, rough drafts of reports, half-finished thought record sheets—you name it. This is problematic because if you are subpoenaed, you may have to forward copies of everything, rough notes and all. As well, despite your best efforts, files can get so thick that you waste a surprising amount of time sifting through them. When the client leaves therapy, you will want to shift the file into your inactive file archive to save space.

So sooner or later you'll be faced with the unpleasant task of going through your files and tossing the surplus into the "to shred" pile. No one likes doing this. And look! Just outside your door, there's your assistant, waiting for the next task. Maybe he can keep you organized.

Resist the temptation to hand the task to your assistant. A colleague of mine once handed a stack of old client files to her assistant to cull. He pulled out everything that looked like handwritten session notes (my friend never had any other kind) and shredded them. Months later the clinician opened an old file to find that all of her session notes were gone. Disaster. And something of an unintentional ethical violation.

Your files are *your* files. They are your responsibility and yours alone. Although it is just fine to delegate some tasks to your assistant, it is your job to make sure client information is handled properly. So unless you have a very experienced assistant who has been thoroughly coached and has shown that he understands how to reorganize or cull your files, do it yourself. You'll sleep easier.

KEEP COMPUTER DATA SECURE

Computers sometimes seem designed to be nonsecure. There are four main sources of security problems for confidential information on computers:

Managing Client Information

- Other people can use your computer and take a look at the files.

- Viruses and related problems can cause your computer to release data over the Internet (through e-mail or by enabling hackers to get access to your files).

- Thieves can simply steal the whole computer, files and all.

- Confidential information can be accessed directly from your backup devices or from the hard drive of some printer-copiers.

All four scenarios are possible, and having someone attempt at least one of them is a virtual certainty sooner or later. You need to ensure effective computer security.

First, get a good virus-detection program and be sure it automatically updates itself. Know, however, that even if your program updates daily, you have only reduced the likelihood of problems. You have not eliminated all risk. You will eliminate the danger only if you keep your office computer free of the Internet and e-mail. It's a good idea, but you aren't likely to do it.

Second, practice good computer hygiene with your office computer. Be cautious about the websites you visit. Dump unsolicited e-mail immediately, and educate everyone in your office against using the business computers for randomly surfing the Web. Be sure everyone knows not to open e-mail attachments unless they are certain of the contents and to consult you if they have any doubts about clicking a link from an e-mail.

Third, store client files on an encrypted flash drive. These are as fast as your hard drive for simple word processing. They are also easy to use, small enough to transport easily, and can—must—be removed at the end of each day and put away in a locked area. This way other people cannot see your confidential files if they use your computer. Viruses remain a problem while the flash drive is attached, but there is a degree of protection against files being broadcast randomly. And thieves may get your machine but not your flash drive, provided you keep it secure. Even if they get the flash drive, they won't have easy access to the files and are unlikely to spend the time trying.

Fourth, be sure any peripheral storage devices (such as backup drives) are encrypted or kept in especially secure storage locations. Check your printer-copier-fax machine to determine whether it has a hard drive that stores information. If so, learn how to clear the memory. Do this regularly, and make especially certain to do it before reselling it or tossing it out.

Is there more? Of course. Take a look at your ethics guide for additional guidelines. These are some of the strategies that have made life easier at my own clinic.

CHAPTER 7

Managing Finances

When private practices fail, it's usually because clinicians dislike thinking of the practice as a business, so they don't run it like one. A business in denial is a business in trouble.

Why aren't people more comfortable with the fact that they are running a business?

- You want to do therapy, not run a business. Every minute you spend working on the financial end of things is a minute away from clinical work.

- You have no training in business. Consequently, business issues are anxiety provoking: *That's not what I'm good at.* This pulls for avoidance, and there are always other things you can think about.

- You're not supposed to be in it for the money. You're doing this out of the goodness of your heart, remember? Focusing on money emphasizes that you are not as charitable as you like to think.

- You have bad associations with receiving immediate payment. People come into your room, you perform a service, and they pay you. The association with other time-honored professions is hard to escape for some therapists.

The fact remains, however, that in private practice you *are* operating a business, a financial venture in which people pay you for what is often an intangible service. Failure to attend to this fact will inevitably lead to problems. So in this chapter let's follow the money.

DON'T LOWBALL YOUR FEE

People contemplating private practice often balk at the recommended fees for therapy: "I'm not worth 150 dollars an hour!" They think back to their last organizational jobs and wonder how they can justify earning two to four times as much.

There's no need: they won't. Consider what you do in the course of a day and whether or not you are paid for that time when you work in a large organization and when you are in private practice (see table 7.1).

Table 7.1 Reimbursement by Activity, Private vs. Salaried Positions

Activity: Are you paid for...?	Large Organization	Private Practice
Preparing for sessions	Yes	No
Writing session notes	Yes	No
Correspondence	Yes	No
Attending meetings	Yes	No
Supervising your assistant	Yes	No

Managing Finances

Marketing	Not needed	No
Planning your services	Yes	No
Reading reports and research	Often	No
Coffee breaks	Yes	No
Chatting with coworkers	Yes	No
Sick time	Yes	No
Vacation and statutory holidays	Yes	No
Working on finances	Yes	No
Seeing clients	Yes	Yes

Clearly when we compare your hourly wage in a traditional workplace with your fee in private practice, we are talking about entirely different things. What about your expenses? Let's compare again with the hourly wage you earn working in a large organization (see table 7.2).

Table 7.2 Expenses Paid from Income, Private vs. Salaried Positions

Expenses: Does your pay have to cover…?	Large Organization	Private Practice
Office lease	No	Yes
Light, heat, telephone, janitorial services	No	Yes
Furniture	No	Yes
Business licenses	No	Yes
Assistant's salary	No	Yes
Office supplies	No	Yes
Printing services	No	Yes

139

Promotional expenses	No	Yes
Waiting-room expenses	No	Yes
Insurance	Not usually	Yes
Workshop fees	Often no	Yes
Retirement plan	No	Yes
Other benefits	No	Yes
Take-home pay	Yes	Yes

So not only do you earn money for less of the time you spend at the office, but also those revenues have to pay for much more than when you work for an organization. All you get to take home is the amount left over after every other bill has been paid. In private practice your *fee* is not your *pay*. Don't confuse the two. Check the fees charged by your colleagues at the same level of training, and consider starting out at a similar rate. A clinician is not a cheap pair of shoes; people don't usually shop for bargains.

CHARGE FOR THE TIME THINGS ACTUALLY TAKE

Recently a member of a local practitioner's e-mail discussion list reported that she had been invited to present a full-day workshop in another city. She asked what people thought she should charge.

Several people suggested that it depended on why she wanted to do the talk. Clinicians often speak on their pet topics at no charge. The reward is having the opportunity to contribute to the profession, advance your point of view, and raise the profile of your practice. It was fairly clear from her post, however, that she wanted public speaking to be a part of her practice, a business venture.

One respondent picked up on this and advised her not to undersell herself, recommending that she charge her usual client rate multiplied by the number of hours in the presentation. This seemed reasonable to some, but let's do the math.

Let's say her usual rate was 150 dollars per therapy hour, and the presentation was seven hours long. That would result in a charge of 1,050 dollars. Not bad, but think of what we're really considering:

- *Presentation time:* Seven hours.

- *Setup and breakdown time:* Usually there are several hours of setup and breakdown time when you do a workshop. Let's be conservative and say just an hour.

- *Travel time:* The conference was a four-hour flight away, meaning there would be a minimum of seven hours of travel each way, resulting in fourteen hours total. We'll presume that the hosts would pay for airfare, hotel, and all other travel expenses.

- *Research and writing time:* Count on a minimum of two hours of preparation for every hour of speaking (ten to one is more realistic, but we'll assume this clinician is fast), so fourteen hours.

- *Audiovisual preparation:* Most talks use presentation software, and we'll assume she decided not to do anything fancy—three hours.

Result: A total of thirty-nine hours spent on the presentation. At the suggested $1,050 fee, this would make a pay rate of $26.92 an hour. This might be fine. Again, sometimes you'll be content to make nothing at all, and in any case not everything you do needs to make the same fee. If the plan is to start a workshop business, however, it is useful to ask yourself whether you are happy with this rate of pay.

Perhaps you don't want to run seminars. The point still applies. Sooner or later you'll be asked to write a report for a lawyer or insurance company. If you're like most people in private practice, you'll finish and think, *Sure, that took four hours. But if I were as smart as I pretend, or as organized as other people surely must be, that report would have taken only half as long. Let's bill for two hours.*

This is reasonable early on, when you're still figuring out your format, but the temptation will be to keep doing this for the rest of your career. We want to be fair to people and not overcharge them. But if we fail to charge properly for our work, we'll undermine ourselves, and the practice—the *business*—will slip from black to red ink. So calculate the time tasks actually take and charge honestly for what you do.

YOUR FIRST FEW CLIENTS ARE TAX FREE

One of the most common ways to start private work is to keep your day job and see a few clients after hours. If you do this, you may have a twinge of discouragement: *Sure, I'll make more money, but I'll pay more taxes too.* Ultimately, yes. But not at first.

If you are employed in a regular salaried position, you have a very limited number of tax deductions: charitable donations, support for dependents, and so on. In some jurisdictions you cannot deduct any significant professional expenses unless you are self-employed.

The tax structure in many countries is designed to allow professionals and entrepreneurs to deduct most or all of the expenses of establishing and operating their businesses. This does not usually depend on the size of the business or the percentage of your income you derive from it. Consequently, someone who sees a single client a week can deduct many of the same amounts as a person who sees twenty-five people a week. If you have a two-hour-per-week practice, you will probably be able to deduct just about all of the income from those clients, with the result that this income is, in effect, tax free. Check with an accountant or tax lawyer, of course, because rules vary by country and state. Washington state, for example, imposes a business and occupation ("B&O") tax on gross receipts, meaning that you pay tax on virtually all earnings before deductions.

Here are some examples of expenses you may be able to deduct from your private practice. Consult an accountant for information about your region.

- Professional fees, such as membership in your profession's regulatory organization

- Professional insurance

- Membership in professional organizations

- Registration fees and travel expenses related to educational workshops and conventions

- Vehicle use for the distance traveled in the service of your business

- Expenses associated with entertaining current or prospective business contacts or customers

- All supplies and furnishings purchased for the business or, in some cases, percentages of these items when they are to be shared between the business and other uses

- Space rental costs

- Books and journals purchased for the business

- A portion of your home's mortgage interest if you have a home office

…and more (or less, depending on where you live).

Can you deduct more than you earn? Ask your accountant, as jurisdictions vary. Most governments recognize that a new business may incur start-up costs that exceed initial revenues, so declaring a loss may be allowable—at least for a while. There must be some hope that the business will eventually earn a profit, so you should not expect to be able to run losses forever without getting audited.

KEEP BUSINESS AND HOME ACCOUNTS SEPARATE

If you incorporate your business (more about that later), you will have to keep the corporation's books separate from your personal finances. If, instead, you maintain your practice as a partnership or sole proprietorship, the rules are somewhat looser. But you should still keep your personal and business books separate.

A ship's compass and charts allow the captain to decide when to change course. In a business, the revenue and expense summaries serve a similar function. If these figures are blended with your household expenses, the performance of the business will be much less obvious to you. You lose basically nothing by separating home and business books, credit cards, and bank accounts. There may be a few more bank charges, but the benefit in keeping everything straight is worth it.

Every month, tally all of your gross business revenues from all sources, within and across all revenue streams (client payments, consulting fees, and so on). Tally all of your business expenses (in and across categories if this proves useful). Then subtract your expenses from the gross revenue to get your net revenue. This is the amount that the business is actually making. Changes in this number month to month, and compared with the same month the previous year (to overcome seasonal effects), tell you more than anything else whether the ship needs to be steered more firmly. Changes in the subsidiary figures (such as the various revenue streams) will give hints about what needs to be done.

PAY YOURSELF A BASE SALARY

One of the disadvantages of private practice is the unpredictability of your income. When revenues are down, you can worry about going broke. When revenues go up, you can relax a little, but you will worry about the next dip. As just discussed, it's a good idea to pay attention to the monthly balance between revenue and expenses. But you can also scale down your anxiety if you inject a bit of predictability into your take-home income.

Take a look at your monthly personal (nonbusiness) expenses (a "Private-Practice Income: Requirements and Projections" worksheet is available at the websites noted in the introduction): your mortgage, your bills, the amount you spend on food and clothing. Don't forget your tax payments. Total it up and add a margin of five to ten percent. This is the amount of money you need to take home each month in order to get by.

Next, look at your practice's net revenues (the income less your business expenses) for the past year. If you are just starting out, take your most pessimistic projections and cut them back by another third. Add any other regular and predictable income sources you have. Estimate the net revenue from all sources that you can fairly confidently rely on each month: "Almost no matter what happens, I can count on making $_____." If possible, trim this figure back by five to ten percent to be even more conservative.

Compare this pessimistic revenue projection with your personal expenses. If the expense total is larger, you're in trouble. Pay special attention to the next section of this chapter. If the revenue total is larger than your expenses, you're in luck: private practice may be workable for you without a major lifestyle adjustment.

What should you pay yourself from the private practice? Your take-home pay (when combined with revenue from other sources) should be a steady monthly check equal to or slightly greater than the minimum survivable income you have identified, but no greater than your pessimistic revenue projection. Keep an eye on the business accounts to be sure what you thought was pessimistic wasn't actually too optimistic.

The result of this system is that your personal income (and thus your self-esteem) won't rise and fall each month based on fluctuations in your practice's revenue. You may not be rich, but you will be able to count on a certain amount of money. If you have been sufficiently conservative in your projections, the amount of money left in your business account each month will creep upward. This is good. You'll have unexpected business expenses now and then, and you will want to have a cushion to handle them.

Every three months, take a close look at the business account. How much has it built up? Does it now hold an amount you will never realistically need? If so, issue yourself a quarterly bonus based not on what you want but on what you have actually brought into the business. This bonus will feel like a treat rather than a necessity. If one quarter the bonus is smaller than the last, well, perhaps it's a seasonal fluctuation. Look at last year's quarterly results to see if you need to change something.

Every year, take another look at your records. Is your revenue reliably exceeding your base paycheck? Are the bonuses getting bigger, and is the reserve fund in the business account growing? If so, consider increasing your monthly paycheck. Conversely, if income is declining (for example, if you are seeing fewer clients so you can work on a book project) and as a result the reserve is shrinking, you might need to shrink your base income—and think about steering the business a bit more firmly.

Let's try it out. Look at the example monthly revenue-minus-expense figures that follow in table 7.3. In the past year, you averaged $4,084.33 per month and made less than $3,000.00 only twice, in June and February. It looks as if you can count on at least $3,000.00 a month after expenses, especially if you plan to leave a buffer of a few thousand dollars in the business account. We'll imagine that your personal expenses total $2,550.00, so a $3,000.00 paycheck each month should be manageable for the coming year.

Table 7.3 Net Income by Month

Month	Revenue Minus Expenses
June	$2,652
July	$3,508

Month	Revenue Minus Expenses
August	$3,267
September	$4,753
October	$4,139
November	$4,362
December	$3,967
January	$4,403
February	$2,894
March	$5,020
April	$4,865
May	$5,182

Table 7.4 shows the result for the next year. Imagine that you start in June with $4,000 in the business account. That month you make $2,946 once you have paid your expenses. Added to the $4,000 you already had in the account, you now have $6,946. You pay yourself the usual $3,000, leaving $3,946 in the account (which appears as the reserve for the following month). In July you make $3,684, so the business account now has $7,630 in it.

In most months you make a bit more than your base salary of $3,000, and the reserve gets larger. By August there is $7,995 in the account, and after paying yourself your monthly $3,000, there is still $4,995 left over. This enables you to issue a conservative quarterly bonus in August of $1,000.

You continue to earn more than the previous year, and in November you can afford a bonus of $2,500. You could manage a higher bonus, but you decide to let the reserve grow a bit. Revenues continue fairly steadily to February, when a vacation cuts revenue almost in half, but you can still afford the $3,000 salary and another $2,500 quarterly bonus.

Table 7.4 Personal Pay and Bonuses by Month

Month	Revenue Minus Expenses	Bank Account Reserve Plus Revenue	Your Pay
June	$2,946	$4,000 + $2,946 = $6,946	$3,000
July	$3,684	$3,946 + $3,684 = $7,630	$3,000
August	$3,365	$4,630 + $3,365 = $7,995	$3,000 + bonus $1,000
September	$4,932	$3,995 + $4,932 = $8,927	$3,000
October	$4,225	$5,927 + $4,225 = $10,152	$3,000
November	$4,691	$7,152 + $4,691 = $11,843	$3,000 + bonus $2,500
December	$4,053	$6,343 + $4,053 = $10,396	$3,000

Month	Revenue Minus Expenses	Bank Account Reserve Plus Revenue	Your Pay
January	$4,636	$7,396 + $4,636 = $12,032	$3,000
February	$2,746	$9,032 + $2,746 = $11,778	$3,000 + bonus $2,500
March	$5,495	$6,278 + $5,495 = $11,773	$3,000
April	$5,284	$8,773 + $5,284 = $14,057	$3,000
May	$5,378	$11,057 + $5,378 = $16,435	$3,000 + bonus $4,000

By May, revenues are ramping up in what seems to be a seasonal busy period, and you can afford a $4,000 bonus. Meanwhile, the reserve has grown to over $9,000. You are reliably making more than your monthly salary, so you can consider giving yourself a raise, perhaps to $3,500 or $3,750, and if revenues keep up, you'll still have enough left over to issue bonuses to yourself.

Aren't you wasting investment opportunities with the rainy day fund? Possibly, but you can also put it into short-term investments. And you never have to panic when revenues take a little dip, you never run out of money, and you always feel just a little wealthy—all by minimizing your salary and making your pay more predictable.

LIVE A MORE FINANCIALLY CONSERVATIVE LIFE

If you work in a salaried position, you know almost to the dollar how much money you will earn every month. You can divide it across various commitments: a mortgage, a car payment, a gym or club membership, a vacation property, and so on. You can live close to the wire because you know exactly where the wire is.

Private practice is less predictable. The phone will stop ringing, and you won't get a referral for three weeks. You'll put your back out and have to take it easy for a month. This would be a disaster if you were committed to spending close to what you earn. Even if your average take-home pay is the same as in your last salaried position, your actual revenue will vary from month to month, and you will have no safety net if the income dips or stops.

So rather than budget your life to within $100 of your pay, create a simpler life, perhaps one that requires $1,000 less than your average take-home pay. Buy a less expensive home, pay a higher down payment when you buy a vehicle, and be much less willing to commit to ongoing expenses.

Sooner or later you get the amount in the reserve business fund anyway. What do you do with all that extra money? Use some of it to compensate for the reduced security involved in owning your own business. Maximize your contributions to your retirement savings plan, pay off all credit cards monthly, accelerate your car payments and other loans, and keep a larger float of money (in a savings account or short-term investments) in case of emergencies or revenue downturns.

Once you have built up that cushion, continue to live a slightly more Spartan existence than a person with the same income in a salaried job, at least in terms of committed monthly money requirements. That may sound dismal, but living without financial stress is a good strategy for creating peace of mind and a more harmonious life. Then start investing, creating a separate revenue stream that's not dependent on clients. You can also use it on expenditures, such as travel, that don't commit you to earning the same amount every month. So compared to people in salaried positions, you might live in a more modest home, but you might travel more widely, see more plays, and ski more often than they would be able to afford. The things you would spend money on would be activities and experiences that are easier to cut back if difficult financial circumstances dictate. The result is more security, less anxiety, and probably a more interesting life.

DON'T BE OPTIMISTIC

When I introduce cognitive therapy to clients, they often say, "Oh, you mean positive thinking." I don't. Positive thoughts can be just as distorted and just as harmful as negative ones. A lot of cognitive therapy involves overcoming unrealistic positive thinking.

Businesses fail largely through positive thinking. Much of this book is about overcoming optimistic distortions of reality: "I don't need to thank my referral sources." "I don't need a website." "I can get by without paying much attention to revenues and expenses."

There is one particular bit of math that our hopeful demon tries to make us do: "Let's see, forty hours in a week. What would I earn if I saw forty clients? Forty times $150 is $6,000. Multiply that by fifty-two weeks and we've got $312,000. Hey, wouldn't that be great?"

This way lies madness. The figure you arrive at becomes your concept of your potential earning power. Anything less than this becomes an underachievement. It is a brilliant way to make yourself miserable and unsatisfied with any other degree of success. The truth is you can never see this many clients in a week or work fifty-two weeks in a year. If you tried, you would provide poor service and burn out. Dissatisfaction is not created by your income alone. It is produced by the contrast between what you have and what you think you should achieve.

Instead, think of the practice you would like to have. Calculate the minimum income you need to get by. Evaluate the business prospects coldly, without sunny optimism. If the prospects meet that minimum level, then get started. If you do this properly, you will have underestimated your revenue. Every inch by which you exceed your projections will be a bonus, a surprise, an exhilarating success.

There is a place for taking risks. Every business owner tosses the dice now and then, and you will too. But there is also a place for sunny optimism. It is called the bankruptcy trustee's office.

THINK ABOUT HAVING A SLIDING SCALE

Many psychotherapists offer a sliding fee scale for clients in difficult financial circumstances. You are not required to have a sliding scale, however. Many people take the view that their fees are based on what the service costs, not on the income of the purchaser. The price of most goods and services in our culture does not depend on the purchaser's buying power.

If you decide to offer a sliding scale, you should define the range. Typically the upper end of your range is your regular fee: the going rate in the community or the fee suggested by your professional organization. You will probably expect most clients to pay this rate.

Does the scale slide down to zero? You can do this, but remember that your fee covers both your salary and your overhead. If your fee is $100 an hour, probably $40 or more of that will go toward your overhead, not into your pocket. The overhead doesn't change when you see a client pro bono. So if you see someone "for free," in effect you may be paying $40 an hour for the privilege.

Consequently, most practitioners charge enough to pay for their overhead and (often) to provide at least some take-home income as well. Usually the lower bound of the sliding scale is 50 percent or more of the full fee. The closer the lowest fee is to your full fee, the less reason there is to offer it at all: it doesn't provide a significant benefit to the client. If you're going to bother with a sliding scale, make the bottom end a significant reduction.

How do you decide what a client should pay? Most clinicians bring up the sliding scale with clients only when circumstances suggest that the cost of service might be a significant consideration. If you raise the subject with everyone, you run the risk of having upper-to-middle-income earners arguing for a fee reduction on the grounds of having exorbitant mortgage payments.

Few clinicians require documentation of reduced financial ability. The usual practice is to take clients' descriptions of their circumstances at their word. Some clinicians have a preprinted card that notes the fee for each of several family income levels; the client simply points to the one that fits. This is an elegant solution that may, unfortunately, imply that the reduced fee is not reduced at all, that it is simply the standard fee for people with that income. You may not get the positive alliance "bounce" you otherwise would. A colleague of mine simply notes the end points of the sliding scale, from the lowest to the standard fee, and invites the client to choose. She reports that no one ever chooses the lowest rate; most who are given the range opt to pay $5 to $10 per session above that.

WATCH YOUR EXPENSES

A mental health practice has a significant advantage over many other professions: there are relatively few capital costs at the outset. Dentists and physicians pay a fortune for equipment and need it all on opening day. We need only some standard furniture. Consequently, there is usually no need to go into much debt to start your business. Avoid overcompensating for not needing a dental chair by overspending on psychometric scoring programs, art for the waiting room, or antique furnishings.

The main problem in a mental health practice is the ongoing overhead: rent, phone bills, supplies, assistant's salary, and so on. These expenses are reasonably constant regardless of the number of clients you see. At the beginning of each month, your fees go toward the bills. Once they are paid, for the rest of the month you earn your take-home pay. Every item of overhead moves that day later in the month, and every dime you spend on pens, paper, and photocopying comes directly out of your pocket. For this reason, you should do what you can to limit your overhead. Be very cautious about adopting new monthly work expenses.

Let's imagine that your gross income (before business expenses) averages $5,000 per month, and your overhead (rent, assistant, and so on) is $3,000 per month. You will take home $2,000 net income, or 40 percent of total revenues. Given the variability of revenue in private practice, some months that might decline to 0 percent or less. If you could reduce your overhead to $2,000 a month, your take-home pay would grow by the same amount, making your net earnings a more attractive 60 percent of total revenue to 40 percent overhead. Economizing on the expense side can pay off just as much as attracting more business.

HIRE AN ACCOUNTANT

> *Nonsense. I've been doing my own taxes since I was a teenager. I'm willing to hire a plumber, a cab driver, and a computer installer, but I'll never stoop to hiring an accountant.*

Every now and then, life tosses you a bone. This is one of them. Don't miss it. If you haven't discovered this secret yet, learn it now: accountants are free—better than free, in fact. The universe pays *you* to get an accountant.

Here's why: almost any accountant will save you more in taxes than he charges to calculate them. An accountant will take your financial records, make sense of them, and calculate the amount of tax you need to pay. The accountant will do it faster than you and find deductions you never could. In the process the accountant will complete one of the chores you probably hate the most.

Let's say your accountant charges $800 to do your taxes. She performs a task that would take you perhaps eight hours. We won't even consider the hours of avoidance beforehand and anxious rumination afterward (*Did I do it right? Will I get audited?*). If you charge $100 an hour to see clients and would rather do that than decipher the tax code, then you will earn $800, which you can then use to pay the accountant's bill. So her services are already free.

But imagine that you do it yourself. Tearing your hair out and straining to the best of your ability, you determine that you owe $27,482 for the year. If you waltz down to the accountant's office to drop it off, she does the job for you and reports that you owe $25,672. You saved $1,810 by not doing a task you hate.

Don't believe me? Ask your colleagues whether they regret hiring an accountant. If you're still not convinced, do your taxes yourself, then take the same records to an accountant. Compare the numbers and deduct the accountant's fee. You will almost certainly find that the accountant saves you money.

Note: you do not need an accountant to add up every revenue and expense. Any spreadsheet program can do that. But for year-end taxes, hiring an accountant is an obvious choice. She will also be able to advise you on other issues, such as sales taxes, the merits of incorporation, and so on.

CONSIDER INCORPORATION

Legislation varies by region and country, but in most areas you have three options for organizing and registering your business: sole proprietorship, joint partnership, and incorporation.

In a sole proprietorship you own the business outright. In effect, you *are* the business. All of the benefits flow directly to you, and you are responsible for all of the expenses and liabilities.

In a joint partnership, you and one or more others own the company jointly. The owners collect the revenues and are responsible for debts. Usually you would have a legal document specifying the percentage of the company each partner owns, what happens if one partner dies, and what happens if one partner wants out of the business. Two partners, each holding 50 percent of the voting rights, can easily deadlock over any issue, tilting you into instant conflict. Even if the two of you are best friends, happily married, or otherwise related in a cheerful and conflict-free relationship, you *must* have a legal document laying down the ground rules of the venture, and you must get this on paper and signed very early in the partnership. If freedom is one of the attractions of private work, it's hard to imagine why you would shackle yourself to someone else voluntarily. I suggest avoiding joint partnerships.

The third option is incorporation (which still gives you the option of owning the company jointly with someone else). Incorporation literally creates a corpus, or body, for your company separate from your own. It turns your business into a kind of legal person, responsible for its own debts.

An incorporated company earns revenue inside the shell of the company, spends money on expenses and investments, pays salaries to its employees (including the owner), and pays dividends out of profits to its shareholders (you and any partners). There are two primary reasons to incorporate a private practice:

- *Tax advantages:* Profits made and kept inside the corporation are usually taxed at a lower rate than money earned by an individual. Once the money leaves the corporation (for example, in salary payable to you), it gets taxed at the personal rate. The tax advantage is really only significant if a large block of revenue will stay inside the company—for example, in the purchase of an office suite or for other investments. If all or almost all the net revenue gets paid to the owner as salary, the benefit is minimal.

- *Liability:* What happens if the business goes into debt or if you are sued for malpractice? In a sole proprietorship you are responsible for the debts of the firm. If you can't pay out of revenue, your creditors can lay claim to your assets, such as your car, your house, and your personal bank accounts. A corporation is responsible for its own debts. People or companies to whom you owe money can go after your company's assets, but your personal assets outside the company are relatively safe. It is for this protection that many health professionals incorporate. You should check with a lawyer or your malpractice insurer, however: in some circumstances (and jurisdictions), the practitioner's own assets are not significantly protected by incorporation.

If you choose to incorporate, consider hiring a lawyer or purchasing a guide to incorporation for small business. The administrative and paperwork burden is actually quite small for a simple business. As of this writing, however, most mental health private practitioners in Canada and the United States choose not to incorporate, because the benefits are relatively small.

REGISTER FOR APPLICABLE TAXES

One of the factors that can make private practice seem daunting is the necessity of dealing with tax issues. If you have been employed by a large organization for some time, you have probably become used to the organization dealing with income and all other taxes for you. In private practice the burden of registering for and paying tax will fall on you.

The problem is not insurmountable, however. Governments genuinely want people to pay their taxes, so they are motivated to make the process as simple as possible. Most tax matters for people with small businesses sound more complicated than they are. Have your accountant help get you set up, and if there is anything unusual about your business, consider consulting a tax lawyer for advice.

Here are a few of the taxes you may have to deal with:

- *Your own income tax:* Depending on your jurisdiction and the type of company (incorporated or proprietorship), you may need to take monthly deductions from your pay or make quarterly tax payments.

- *Payroll taxes for your employees:* If you have assistants, they will be paid biweekly or monthly and may need to have income tax and various other items deducted from their pay. There may be regulations about the type of health benefits you must include, and you might wish to set up additional benefits for your employees.

- *Goods and services or value-added taxes:* Sales taxes at the municipal, provincial, state, or federal level may or may not apply to the various activities for which you bill. Some professions or types of service are exempted from collecting tax; others are not. Some schemes (such as Canada's GST) allow registrants to deduct the tax they have paid out to suppliers from the tax payable to the government.

- *Workers' compensation:* Some regions require that employers pay premiums for what are, in effect, insurance programs for workers who may be injured on the job. This may apply to everyone associated with your practice (including you), or it might be limited to your assistant. Because office work typically entails a minimal risk of injury, the premiums are usually quite low for people in these job categories.

- *Business licenses:* Some municipalities require that you take out an annual license to carry on a business within the boundaries of the town.

There may be other forms of tax in your area. Ask your accountant for guidance.

SET UP YOUR OWN RETIREMENT PLAN AND BENEFITS

In private practice you have the choice of doing without benefits or, better, arranging them yourself. For simplicity's sake, let's divide these benefits into two parts: retirement savings plans and everything else.

Let's start with "everything else." Some benefits, such as sick days, are simply not available to you. You'll get sick anyway, you'll have to cancel your clients, and you'll cope. The benefits that may apply include health insurance, short-term disability, long-term disability, dental services, and life insurance. If you live in the United States, you will certainly want to purchase health insurance, and it will be a significant expense.

Suppliers of other benefits have noticed the increasing number of people working independently, and they recognize this as a large untapped market. Consequently, many firms now offer benefits packages to private practitioners. Some of these companies offer the package by affiliating with a professional organization, such as a local psychological association. The members of the group can access the service at a reduced cost. Other packages are unaffiliated with any group.

I recommend checking with your professional organization about the availability of a benefits package. Read up on the benefits provided and any limitations on the service (such as a lack of coverage for disability caused by preexisting conditions). Then consider your own life circumstances. If you don't absolutely require an income, or if you have few fixed expenses or no dependent children or elders, it may be less useful for you to subscribe to one of these programs. If a period of disability would be catastrophic for you, then financial security is more of an issue. One option is to subscribe to a benefits package. Another is to maintain regular employment for as many days per week as are required to stay on the organizational benefits plan.

What about retirement plans? If you take the optimistic view that your federal government pension plan will provide for you in your later years, you need to rethink: funding of these plans is highly suspect and may not be there when you need it. Perhaps you imagine, based on your ancestors' limited life spans, that you will never need a plan. This "optimistic pessimism" is likewise suspect. You cannot rely on that familial heart problem, genetic disorder, or accident proneness to be your retirement plan.

Instead, you need to plan ahead for yourself. Get to the bank, your accountant, or a reputable financial planner, and put a savings plan in place. For most people the only strategy that really works is to have the funds automatically transferred from their bank account to their retirement account—RSP, 401(k), or SEP-IRA—on a monthly basis. You never see the money, so you can't spend it on anything else. Don't think you could cut much out of your budget? David Chilton's excellent and readable investing book *The Wealthy Barber* (1989; subsequently revised) asserts that if you deduct 10 percent of your after-tax income automatically from your account—an amount that can seem huge and unaffordable—within two months you will never miss it, and your lifestyle will not be noticeably affected.

If you have not yet started a retirement savings plan, do so now. Do not wait for your mortgage to be paid off, your children to grow up, your credit-card balance to be zero, or your horoscope to declare today an excellent day for retirement planning. And do not rely on your own self-discipline, striving daily to save money so you will have a chunk to put into your retirement plan. Start an automatic withdrawal system, and then ramp it up as much as you can. If you discover that you can't live on what's left, what have you lost? You still have all that money, and you can always take it out again.

※

If you take the sober steps in this chapter seriously, you will run your practice in full recognition of what it truly is: a business. If you fail to treat the financial side seriously, you will not be in practice for long.

Come up with some good questions based on the particulars of your practice and your country, state, or province. Take them to your accountant or to a good tax lawyer. Get the right answers and put them into practice. Then start helping people. You'll help more of them this way, and you'll do it for more years than if you attempt to ignore financial realities.

CHAPTER 8

The Clinic Assistant

A friend of mine operates a bedding store in a trendy area of Vancouver. A travel magazine once listed buying sheets at his store as one of the top five things to do in the city. So the place is successful, but Tuesdays are slow. Rather than hire someone for those days, he staffs the store himself and does his own paperwork and mail orders. It's an efficient solution to the problem of an empty store.

Similarly, when you start out in a practice, you may have plenty of slack time while you're waiting for the phone to ring. Rather than morosely surf the Internet, you can do all of the clinic chores: photocopy handouts, research possible referral sources, answer the phone, type practice documents, handle billing, and so on. As the practice gets busier, the number of these nonclinical tasks increases, and the time left over to accomplish them decreases. The resulting anxiety is your signal that it's time to think about hiring an assistant. Let's consider the basics.

CALCULATE THE HOURS YOU NEED

Unless you have a bustling multiple-clinician practice, you may never need a full-time assistant. You won't see so many people that the hours of paperwork exceed the hours of clinical contact. So if you hire an assistant, the person will most likely work part-time. How many hours do you need? Let's work it out (a "Calculation Form for Your Clinic Assistant's Hours" is available at the websites noted in the introduction):

1. Estimate the number of hours of administrative or clerical work the clinic generates in a week (whether or not you actually manage to complete it all): _____.

2. How many hours of this work will you have to or want to keep doing yourself, even if you get an assistant? _____ (Don't answer, "None"; you will never get away from clinic management tasks completely, and there is something soothing about doing tasks that don't require too much mental effort.)

3. Subtract step 2 from step 1. This is the number of hours of work that you could give someone else to do: _____.

4. Multiply step 3 by 1.25, in light of the fact that your assistant will probably take more time than you at many tasks, and because your practice will grow a bit more when your own time is freed up: _____.

5. Multiply step 3 by 1.75, which is a more generous estimate of the hours the assistant's job will occupy: _____.

6. Estimate how much you will pay the assistant per hour: _____.

7. Multiply step 6 by step 4: _____ and multiply step 6 by step 5: _____. This tells you approximately how much your assistant will cost under both the conservative and liberal estimates.

8. Divide step 7 by the hourly fee you charge to see clients.

   step 6 × step 4 / rate = _____

   step 6 × step 5 / rate = _____ .

You have just calculated the number of extra hours you will need to see clients each week to pay for your assistant. Though approximate, the figures are close enough to give you a hint what the costs would be. What most people discover is that they can buy between five and twelve hours of help by adding just one more hour of clinical work. And by handing off all of that paperwork to an assistant, they would free up more than enough time to do so. If you have enough referrals, you can earn more and spend fewer hours at the clinic, while getting rid of tasks that detract from the reason you opened the practice in the first place.

If this looks like a good trade-off, consider hiring someone for the number of hours calculated in step 5 or, if you are still uncertain, step 4.

MAKE ROUTINE THINGS ROUTINE

Every business can expect the unexpected now and then, and some tasks or situations come up only once in a decade. Most things that happen in a private practice, however, happen with some frequency. People call and want to see a therapist. A bill needs to be created. A client's check bounces. Someone needs a duplicate receipt for a payment made last year.

The simplest thing to do with any task is to improvise a solution on the spot. Type a new receipt. Improvise a bill. Grab a piece of paper and jot down the referral details. It would take two to five times as long to come up with an organized system for carrying out the task.

For repetitive tasks, however, having a system in place will cut the time markedly. Rather than type all the details of a bill, you'll just have to open the billing file and fill in a few boxes. Eventually you'll save more time than it took you to develop the system.

Consider a chore that takes 15 minutes to complete, like improvising a thank-you letter for a recent referral. Imagine that it would take 45 minutes to develop a template for generating such a letter and that once you have a system in place, it would take you 5 minutes each time. The first time you create a letter, improvising is clearly more efficient: 15 versus 45 minutes. The second time, improvising is still preferable: 30 minutes (2 × 15) versus 50 minutes (45 + 5). By the fourth time, the time spent creating the system is balanced by the time saved: 60 minutes each. By the tenth time, the system takes 90 minutes, whereas doing the chore without a system takes 150 minutes. If the problem comes up once a week, by year-end you will have saved an eight-hour workday by spending 45 minutes coming up with a system. You don't need many of these systems to begin saving huge chunks of your time.

So if you ask, "What's the fastest way of doing this?" the answer depends on whether you mean *this* time or long term. For almost all routine tasks, the answer is that spending the time to develop a routine way of handling the situation is eventually faster. The more routine a task is, the easier it will be for assistants to learn how to handle it, and the less often they will have to consult you for clarification. Your own time saved may be close to 100 percent. Consequently, when you contemplate hiring an assistant, it is worthwhile to spend a lot of extra time creating standard routines for the tasks the assistant will be asked to undertake.

Which tasks should be a priority for this systematizing? The answer is obvious: those that recur most often, and those for which having a system will produce the greatest time saving per occasion. Don't waste too much time deciding between the options, however, because almost no matter what you choose, you will be spending your time well. Once you have systematized the obvious tasks, your ongoing job will be to create systems for the remaining chores, perhaps with your assistant's help.

HAVE A CLINIC MANUAL

Systems are irrelevant if no one knows what they are. It's easy to think you will come up with a way of handling billing, discuss it with your assistant, and be done with it. But you will have to do the chore yourself when your assistant is on vacation. You will have to teach every new assistant you hire, and most people need things explained more than once before they master a new system. As well, once you have taught a system to your assistant, it may be a year before you need to think about it again—and at that point, if you haven't documented it, you will spend as much time trying to recall the system as it took you to set it up the first time.

Consequently, once you have come up with a way of doing things, you should write it down in clear and concise language. Put the resulting guidelines in a bound clinic manual accessible to everyone in the office.

Who should write this manual? Your assistant. Each time the two of you discuss a new system, ask the assistant to write up a draft of the strategy. Proof it for clarity and accuracy—partly to see if you and your assistant have the same understanding of the system, and partly to see if a new staff member could follow the instructions if that's all the person had to go on. Whenever you get a new colleague or assistant, assign reading the manual as a first task.

NEVER HIRE FRIENDS

We are not married to our friends. If they are financially irresponsible, disorganized, slow to return phone calls, occasionally insensitive, or if they dress outlandishly, no problem. Indeed, our friends' eccentricities can help us to stretch our own equanimity and to see life from wildly different points of view.

Employees differ from friends in several respects: you are around them much more often than most friends; you are in a supervisory relationship with them, rather than the equal relationship that friendship ideally strives toward; and you need employees to perform duties in specific ways and cannot afford to adopt the laissez-faire attitude you might have with most friends.

Consequently, transferring from a friendship relationship to an employment relationship is fraught with peril. Just as you should never lend money to a friend unless you are prepared not to get it back, you should not employ a friend unless you are willing to lose the friendship. Consider the ways things can go wrong:

- *Role resistance:* Once we attain equality with another person, we tend to resist losing parity and adopting a subservient role. Despite recognizing that you are the employer, friends will almost certainly chafe in the role in a way that they would not if they had no prior relationship with you. You will tell them what you want them to do much more often than you would have any right to do as a friend, which will begin to grate on them.

- *Presumed capacity:* We tend to see our friends as being like ourselves. You might assume that your friends can write letters, speak in a professional manner on the telephone, maintain confidentiality, cope with insurance company forms, examine contracts and orders for flaws, ritualistically clean and organize the waiting room, and so on. After all, you could do all of these things; surely they can too. But you will always have some rude surprises—and once you have hired a friend, it is too late to do much about it.

- *Employer fantasies:* Just as you have a fantasy about how your friends would be as employees, they will have fantasies about what it would be like to work with you. These fantasies will almost certainly be dashed. Your friend may not believe or fully appreciate any cautions you offer but will quickly discover that you are not as calm or organized as you let on, you make decisions and reverse them minutes later, you ask for input and then do the opposite, you say you get "tense" when you really mean "startlingly irritable," and sometimes working for you is really no fun at all. Disillusionment will set in quicker with you, for whom your friends had such high hopes, than it would for an identical employer they had never met.

- *Supervisory resistance:* Just as your friend may resist taking a one-down position, you may resist adopting a one-up position: "We're all equals here; we just have different jobs." Yes, but someone still has to be the boss, decide what those jobs are, and make final decisions—and that's you. You may become apologetic or anxious about giving your assistant tasks, particularly tasks you don't enjoy. But that, of course, is one of the main reasons for hiring an assistant: so someone else will do the things that you don't like or that don't employ your clinical skills.

- *Termination anxiety:* If an assistant doesn't work out, you can always choose to end the person's employment. But how do you fire a friend? Letting a friend go without damaging the relationship is a very tricky proposition. In effect, no matter how good the person is, you will feel stuck with him. You rely on your friend to live up to your expectations.

Having a friend in an ongoing assistant's position is inherently tricky, but the risks are reduced if you have an extremely defined task and an explicit end date. If you have a large mailing to do and hire your financially distressed friend to stuff envelopes, things will probably be fine. If your friend is a tax lawyer and you want to get specific advice about an issue, you can accept the risk that her advice will be poor or that she will charge more than you expect.

While we're on the topic, your friends may offer to help you with various tasks (setting up your wireless network, creating a revenue spreadsheet) for a reduced or waived fee. Should you accept? Consider your ability to reciprocate. You cannot ethically see your friend as a counseling client, no matter what the issue is or how many favors you owe the person. So don't take a discount from friends for anything having to do with your clinical work.

DON'T DO YOUR ASSISTANT'S JOB

A task is like a possession. Once you give it to your assistant, that person owns it. You are the boss and can take it back if you wish—but not without consequences.

There are several messages you might inadvertently give to an assistant if you perform duties you initially assigned to him: "This workplace is unpredictable and uncontrollable." "Having observed your struggles with this task, I have concluded that you will never learn it." "You don't own anything; nothing in this office is yours, not even the smallest of roles." Each of these messages is discouraging or demoralizing to receive and can contribute to your assistant's job dissatisfaction. The more dissatisfied he is, the less effective he will become and the more likely he will be to seek work elsewhere.

Consequently, think carefully before you hand over any task to an assistant. It is much easier to give responsibility than to take it back, so delegate with forethought. Are you confident that your assistant can perform the task or learn it if need be? Are you content to cede some control? Are you prepared to spend the time necessary to help your assistant master the task?

One way to create problems is to hand your assistant a multi-part task (such as keeping track of your revenues), thinking you will see how much she feels comfortable doing. Then you can check the person's work, leave her with the bits she is good at (such as entering checks into your spreadsheet), and take over the parts she doesn't do well (such as calling clients whose payments are overdue). This seems like a logical way of doing things, but the implied compliment ("You've done well with this part") is overshadowed by the implied criticism ("You're lousy at this other bit"), making the overall experience a negative one for the assistant.

A better strategy is to tease apart complicated tasks you'd like to delegate, identify pieces you are confident the assistant can learn to perform well, and hand those over while continuing to do the rest yourself. Once your assistant has mastered those tasks, add another bit at a time. This way the implied message is repeatedly, "You're good at this; here's something else I'm confident you can do."

Another problem arises when a task seems so trivial that you say to yourself, *Oh, I'll just do this myself rather than wait*; for example, entering a large payment into your revenue system so you can take it to the bank. This is confusing for the assistant, causing more problems than it solves: *Where'd this come from? Have I lost this huge check somewhere? I'd better hunt around here before I ask Dr. Bigshot about it; otherwise I'll look like an idiot.*

Doing tasks for the assistant is usually an unintended show of disrespect, not an improvement in efficiency: *I'll take back part of your job without even bothering to tell you about it.* As well, your assistant may become less diligent about doing the task: *What's the point in checking the mail? It's probably already been done.* It's a bad idea to set up a situation where someone is, in effect, rewarded for being neglectful: *If I don't bother, someone will do it for me.*

So think carefully before handing duties over to an assistant, because they are costly to take back. Once you have handed off a duty, resist the impulse to do it yourself, no matter how easy it might be. If, on the odd occasion, you have no choice but to do so, make a point of apologizing. The clinic may be your business, but you have trespassed on your assistant's territory.

RAISES ARE CHEAPER THAN TURNOVER

Once you have a good assistant, do what you can to keep the person on staff. If you don't give your assistant raises based on performance, he will eventually move on.

But what if your assistant does leave? It's tempting to think that your clinic is not too difficult to run, so training a new person shouldn't be very time consuming. Remember, however, that all of the time you spend replacing someone is calculated at your rate of pay, not your assistant's. Take the example of a clinician who charges $150 an hour to see clients and loses a fifteen-hour-per-week assistant who is paid $15 an hour. What are the costs of turnover?

Developing and posting an online job ad: one hour of your time, billed at $150.

Reviewing and short-listing résumés: two hours, or $300.

Interviewing and deciding among applicants: four hours, or $600.

Perhaps the new person can be partly trained by the outgoing assistant. You will never avoid the task completely, however. Estimate it conservatively at 10 hours of your time, or $1,500.

The total time for the new assistant to learn the job will be twice that, so let's say 20 hours total at her rate of pay, or $300 ($15 per hour × 20 hours).

You will also have to pay your outgoing assistant for those 10 hours he spends training the new assistant, so that's $150.

Imagine that you've been happy with your outgoing assistant. Let's guess that the odds the new person will be as good are fifty-fifty. If she is not as good, let's say she produces only 75 percent as much value as your outgoing assistant. In a year of 15 hours per week, less two weeks of holidays, you will pay 15 hours × 50 weeks × $15 per hour, or $11,250.00. If there's a 50 percent chance of getting only 75 percent as much work from the new assistant, let's calculate this roughly as $11,250 × 50 percent × 25 percent = $1,406.25.

What's the total? The ad ($150) plus the short listing ($300) plus the interviewing ($600) plus the training time for you ($1,500), the new assistant ($300), and the old assistant ($150) plus the lost efficiency ($1,406.25): $4,406.25.

What if a raise could have retained your previous assistant for just one more year? If the cost of taking on a new person is $4,406.25, you could have given your assistant a $5.87 per hour raise, which might have kept that person with you. And if you offered a raise and the assistant quit anyway, you wouldn't have to pay it—so there is no real gamble.

You might quibble about some of the numbers in this example, though they are quite conservative. The point, though, is that giving a raise may seem expensive, but actually it is usually cheaper than replacing a good employee. Raises are not the only way of retaining staff, obviously, but they are one such tool and should not be overlooked.

What kind of raise should you give? It should not be so small that it is insulting or trivial, and it should not be so large that you can't afford to offer raises with some frequency. My preference is to give raises that are as small as possible without going below the first threshold—not to save money, but so I can give raises more often.

It's best that raises be tied to performance rather than simple longevity in the position. If a new hire seems extremely promising, for example, you could give the person a raise after the first month's work. He will not expect this, and it will reinforce the fact that you value his contribution. If you take an extended vacation and things go well in your absence, you might give your employee a raise on your return. You can also provide raises as the assistant takes on additional responsibility (such as managing payroll or updating the clinic's website).

TAKE THE BOSS'S SEAT

There is an inherent power imbalance in employer–employee relationships. One person gets to make the critical decisions, set the priorities, and, when necessary, specify how and when things get done. Ideally this is done with consultation, welcoming the contributions of all staff and implementing useful ideas while giving credit where it is due. But there is a boss's seat, and someone needs to sit in it.

Therapists are often reluctant to occupy the boss's chair. We don't see ourselves as having any right to tell others what to do, we don't want to be perceived as controlling, and most of us want desperately to be liked. We think if we hire someone, we will be "good employers": respectful, consultative, fair, and open to feedback. Good. But this often translates into a reluctance to fulfill the employer role in the relationship.

The resistance to the employer role can manifest in many ways: indecisiveness about task priorities; a misguided desire to be "fair" (such as trying to answer the phone just as often as the person you hired to answer the phone); failure to give corrective feedback on timeliness or work quality; or a reluctance to state clearly what you want in terms of staff work hours, vacation days, and lunch breaks. You gradually build up resentment at the employee's failure to read your mind or guess what you want.

As an employee in my younger years, I found myself annoyed with an employer who was so timidly "fair" and "respectful" that I had no idea what was expected in the job. I wanted to march into my supervisor's office and shout, "Look, I'm here to work, not guess why you hired me! You obviously want me to do something; just tell me what it is, and I'll go do it. And if I can't figure it out, I'll come back and ask!"

As a supervisor I have caught myself being shyly reluctant to tell a new employee that her perpetual lateness was a problem, that hiding unpaid bills in a desk drawer was not acceptable, and that the street address on an envelope should go below the addressee's name, not above it. On the one occasion when I clearly needed to fire someone, I delayed for over a month, hoping the person would realize the job was not for her and quit, thus relieving me of the task.

You don't have to be the office tyrant, but you do need to recognize that as an employer, you have certain responsibilities, and you will be a worse boss, not a better one, if you ignore them. While leaving room for negotiation and discussion, these responsibilities include:

- Stating clearly the hours of the job, the nature of breaks, and the way lunch breaks are handled

- Assigning regular duties and providing clear positive or corrective feedback on the employee's performance

- Specifying how you want things done in a clear and straightforward manner, without ambiguity or dithering

- Assigning additional projects, making the employee's role clear, and providing feedback on performance

- Being absolutely reliable in the timing and accuracy of payroll

Far from being offensive, if you occupy the role you have defined for yourself in the act of hiring, taking your seat as a responsible, communicative employer will help your staff, provide a needed hand on the tiller of the business, and enable you to realize the goals you had in hiring staff in the first place.

DON'T APOLOGIZE FOR ASSIGNING WORK

You hire staff for a reason: there are tasks you don't have time to do or simply don't like to do. Once you have people on staff, you systematically delegate these tasks to them. Because many clinicians have overactive superegos, handing a repetitive or undemanding task to an employee can induce guilt. Clinicians sometimes cope by apologizing profusely for requesting that the person carry out the task: "I know it's not very interesting, kind of drudge work really, very much beneath you, but somebody has to do it and I just don't have the time. I'm so sorry..."

The intent is to seek absolution from the employee for the sin of handing him a task. But giving tasks to your staff is your job; it is why you hired them. If it were not for these tasks, they would not be employed. The unintended and often unperceived effect of the employer's groveling is that the assistant feels belittled: *I don't really mind doing it, but I wish Dr. Genius didn't put the job down so much; she makes me feel kind of insignificant for spending my time on this stuff.*

Don't try not to feel the apologetic temptation, if you are prone to it. Welcome it and review the reality of the situation. Is the task outside the boundaries of the job? If so (it isn't your assistant's job to pick up your dry cleaning), then do not ask her to do it. If the request is reasonable, however, resist the apology. Do not put down the task; do not promise her something more interesting to do tomorrow; do not adopt a pleading, groveling expression. Simply hand your assistant the task in a straightforward manner. If you think she would be more comfortable with an accommodation, suggest it: "I don't have any more appointments this afternoon; feel free to spread out the paper in the waiting room if that helps." "This might be a good job to do with the music system turned up if you like."

PRACTICE AN EFFECTIVE FEEDBACK RATIO

Therapists should be great employers: they combine training in relationships with knowledge of reinforcement theory. Sadly, we often forget to use the principles our own field developed. There are two concepts to remember here.

First, reinforcement is more powerful than criticism as a change strategy. Indirectly, it also cements the relationship, and it helps the receiver feel more confident and able to handle other tasks. By contrast, punishment or harsh criticism seldom leads to more effective behavior unless the feedback giver practices corrective feedback rather than criticism (see the following section). The person who is criticized tends to withdraw, resent the message, attribute the feedback to the critic (*He's a butthead*) rather than to her own performance, and feel less capable of taking on other tasks. The key to improving an employee's performance is to find and comment on the parts of the task the person has done correctly—generally *before* identifying the parts that could have been done better.

Second, criticism is more memorable than praise. Give the average person an employee evaluation that contains both positive and negative comments about his performance, then test his recall. Negatives will usually be recalled with greater accuracy, and the recipient will have the sense of being criticized more than praised. Negative comments seem to be perceived and retained more strongly than positive ones. We could speculate about the reasons, but perhaps we can simply jump to a conclusion: it is not enough for us to praise as much as we criticize. To make up for the psychological heft of negative feedback, we need to balance it out with a larger amount of positive feedback.

How much larger? Psychologist Barbara Fredrickson has examined the effects of positive and negative feedback on functioning (summarized in Fredrickson & Losada, 2005, and in her recent book *Positivity*, 2009) and concludes that a ratio of approximately three positives to one negative produces a higher level of functioning than a ratio nearer parity. If valid, this would support praising employees three or more times as much as we point out failings. Doing so may enable them to open up to corrective feedback. A diet of complete positivity does not seem to be the goal, because it could lead to the feedback giver being dismissed as an irrelevant cheerleader rather than a source of valued information.

WORD CORRECTIVE FEEDBACK EFFECTIVELY

The way we word a correction to an assistant can have a significant impact on whether it solves the problem at hand; whether it causes the person to stay oriented to the task rather than to his own wounded ego; and whether the assistant maintains a positive working relationship with us. Every employee we ever hire will have difficulties and make mistakes, despite our best hopes. As a result, we need to employ strategies for providing corrective feedback effectively (as discussed in *The Assertiveness Workbook*, Paterson, 2000):

Focus on the event, not the person. The point of giving feedback to your assistant is to enable a more effective approach to the task at hand. Anything that causes the person to focus on her own sense of inadequacy is a mistake. We cannot change our long-standing personality traits at will, so there is little point in getting feedback about them from our employers. Instead, receiving feedback that is clearly tied to observable behavior enables us to plan a new way of approaching the task: "When the telephone rings, I'd like you to..." "Instead of putting the agency's name after the postal code, I'd like you to..."

Don't hint. Our discomfort at giving corrective feedback may lead us to avoid addressing the issue directly: "Oh, this is how you've done it? Oh, I'd thought—um, well, this should do—I guess." Hinting inadvertently communicates your dissatisfaction but fails to point out what you wanted done differently or how the person could do it. The assistant gets only the least useful bit of the feedback, which is your emotional reaction to his work. He may try to figure out whether you are really dissatisfied or only distracted, and if the former, then what it might have been that displeased you. He may even try to correct the situation based on his guess, potentially making things even worse if the guess isn't accurate.

Talk one to one. Give praise publicly; provide corrective feedback privately. If you point out problems in front of others, the assistant's attention will invariably be divided between focusing on your words and watching or wondering about the audience's reaction. You will get a larger share of her attention if no one else is present.

Include the positive in the message. When you start giving someone negative feedback, it is never clear how far you will go. Your assistant may wonder if you hate everything she's doing, particularly if she has an overactive internal critic: *As a matter of fact, I haven't liked anything you've done since January.* Be sure to include positive feedback about the aspects that are going well: "Your telephone manner is terrific: warm, professional, attentive. But it would be better to make sure to pick up the phone before the third ring." You can also start by providing a frame around the problem, showing the limits of the criticism before you give it: "This project is working very well, and overall I'm happy. I'd like to increase the proofreading accuracy, though."

Be precise. Our own sense of dissatisfaction is often vague, and we can be tempted to communicate this vagueness to staff without doing the work of narrowing down and specifying the problem: "Dominic, I'd like you to tighten up the referral process" is not helpful; it gives Dominic no information to act on. If he pays attention at all, he will waste a great deal of time trying to decipher the message you are trying to send. You are ready to provide feedback only once you have a clear idea of what's troubling you: "Dominic, I got a call today from a client who thought she was on the waiting list, but she isn't. I'd like for us to sit down and figure out how to keep all of the referrals on track." This communicates the nature of the problem and an intent to work collaboratively on a solution.

Dwell on what you want, not what you don't want. One way of taking the sting out of corrective feedback is to word it in a way that states the goal you want to strive for, rather than the deficiencies you see: "I'd like to be sure print orders go out the week they are received" is better than "You often seem to leave orders sitting for four weeks." You don't have to avoid the current problem, but it often works better if it isn't the first thing out of your mouth. If the staff member responds, "That's what I aim for too," you can say, "Several orders lately have waited four weeks; let's figure out how to shorten that to one."

In summary, once your practice is thriving, you could probably benefit from adding an assistant's hourly wage to your overhead, provided this enables you to conduct a few more billable hours and go home a little earlier. Finding a good assistant is difficult, so once you have one, do what you can to keep her. Systematize routine tasks and hand them off bit by bit to the assistant. Recognize and reinforce effective job performance frequently, and give corrective feedback sparingly, specifically, and constructively. And however daunting this task of staff management might seem, remember that you are an educated health care professional with a specialization in human behavior. If anyone can master this, you can.

CHAPTER 9

Managing Clinical Services

So you've found your space, you've set it up, you've corresponded with referral sources, you've developed your website, you've set up information and financial management systems, you're dressed properly, and your assistant sits in the adjoining office. You're set. There's just something missing. Hmm, what could it—oh, yes: the client.

The point of having a private practice is to deliver services to the public. This imposes the question of how best to organize and provide those services in a sustainable and efficient manner. We will not overconcern ourselves here with the content of your service, whether it is executive coaching, schizophrenia treatment, or educational assessment; whether you use cognitive behavioral therapy, narrative techniques, or sandbox play. Let's treat the nature of your service as a closed package, a black box, but consider how best to structure the delivery of that package. This, then, is the FedEx chapter.

We will start with the creation of a clinical schedule, discuss some ways of clarifying why the client is in your office and the project you will soon embark on, present some methods for making the most of what can seem like an agonizingly short contact, and conclude with some strategies for making the system work over the longer term.

PLAN YOUR CLINICAL WEEK

When you open a practice, you may be so thrilled to get referrals that you will see them just about anytime. As your practice fills, you need to break this precedent and begin planning your week to suit yourself. Balance the demands of the business with your life interests.

Perhaps you dislike racing into the office first thing on Monday morning. Then don't do it. Monday morning isn't prime time for clients anyway. Maybe you like the idea of offering sessions one evening a week so you can afford to take Wednesdays off. Fine. Plan the week around this, and make sure you can come in late the next morning. You like to ski Thursday evenings? Terrific. Plan to leave at 3:00 p.m. every Thursday. You hate seeing clients late on Friday afternoon? It's easily avoided.

Perhaps you don't plan to see clients five days a week. No one ever decreed that you have to do this. If you don't, you can even make a bit of money by renting out your space for the days you aren't there.

Once you have the week blocked out for clinical time, reflect on the number of sessions you can offer per day and per week. Most clinicians have a maximum number of people they can see each day (usually between four and seven), above which they do not function well. They might occasionally book one client more than their maximum, knowing that often there will be a cancellation. Avoid booking your "max-plus-one" more than one day in a week. Sometimes everyone will show up, and now and then you might even get a call from a client in crisis who needs to be seen right away. You can't often exceed your maximum without suffering the effects.

Then consider your appointment times. If you see people for the fabled fifty-minute hour, you could schedule your afternoon with people at one, two, three, and four o'clock. This is a poor idea, however. You need breaks to recover and collect yourself, and if any appointment runs long, it will bump all the others, making you late for the rest of the day. Consequently, it is a good policy not to set more than two appointments in a row back to back.

Here's a sample schedule: Appointment 1 is at 9:00 a.m., allowing you to get to work at 8:30 and settle in before seeing anyone. Appointment 2 is at 10:00, then you have a fifteen-minute break before appointment 3 at 11:15. If either of your earlier appointments runs long, you can still start the third one on time. Lunch is 12:15 to 1:00 p.m., when appointment 4 begins, followed by appointment 5 at 2:00. Then there's another break, shifting appointment 6 to 3:15. Then your energy may be flagging, so you might need another break, pushing appointment 7 to 4:30 (a popular time for clients who want to get off work a bit early and see you at the end of their day). One night a week you may want to open a few slots for working clients, so perhaps your schedule that day will be 1:00 p.m., 2:00 p.m., 3:15 p.m., 4:30 p.m., 5:30 p.m., dinner, 7:15 p.m., 8:15 p.m.

Establishing regular times like this can enable your assistant to book clients for you rather than having to consult with you every time. You can also specify a daily maximum. You could circle up to eight appointment times on the clinic calendar, but write "Max 5" or "Max 6" at the top of the page, so they don't all get filled. Some days you will have other projects to finish, and you can lay out the same number of appointment times but specify "Max 3."

SET STANDARD ASSESSMENT TIMES

When will you see your new clients? One reasonable option is to call them up, find out what time works best for them, and juggle everything else to accommodate them. If you have a new practice without many clients, this may work well.

More frequently, clinicians set aside specific times for assessments. Some have one or two standard assessment slots each week. This system makes it easy for your assistant to keep track of bookings and the waiting list. She can just fit people into the next available slot, whenever it happens to be. This also minimizes the risk of booking a new assessment into a slot that an ongoing client likes to have.

Another system is to look at your schedule every few weeks and decide whether you have room for new clients. Then you can set aside one or more assessment slots and make them available for the next caller or the next person on the waiting list. At my clinic each clinician identifies new assessment slots by circling times in the master appointment book in the assistant's office and writing a circled "A" beside those times. This makes it easy for the assistant to flip through the book while on the phone with a prospective client to see which clinicians are taking new clients and when slots are available.

Many clinicians schedule their assessments at less popular times than their ongoing therapy slots, perhaps midmorning or midafternoon. Most people can put themselves out for one awkwardly timed appointment but will welcome the chance to set ongoing appointments at more convenient times. When booking an assessment, both clinician and assistant should make clear that when the switch is made to ongoing therapy, you will attempt to work out a regular time slot that will work well for both client and provider.

SCHEDULE ASSESSMENTS FOR LONGER THAN USUAL

Throughout my career I have been poor at sticking to the fifty-minute hour when conducting assessments. I never get through all the content I want to cover. This isn't surprising. Think of all the things you want to accomplish in an assessment:

- Make sure you have all the necessary demographic information.

- Review the limits to confidentiality.

Managing Clinical Services

- Secure a release to discuss the case with the client's physician or another professional.

- Establish a warm therapeutic relationship.

- Diagnose the presenting problem.

- Understand the risk factors contributing to the problem.

- Get a sense of the client's corresponding strengths.

- Look for comorbid conditions.

- Take a basic medical history.

- List current medications being taken.

- Score, interpret, and provide feedback on any psychometric instruments.

- Find out about the client's current life situation.

- Sketch the client's background and basic life history.

- Get a feel for the client's interpersonal style and presentation.

- Learn about the previous treatment history and the client's own coping strategies.

- Assess the client's motivation for change.

- Help the client understand that treatment will involve a great deal of work, almost all of which he will do, and much of which will be done between sessions.

...and more.

The reality? You're not going to get through all this. Much of it will have to wait until the second (or third) session, and parts of it (the list of risk factors, understanding the client's strengths, learning about the person's history) will go on for the duration of treatment.

One option is to limit the initial assessment session to the usual fifty minutes, and stretch the assessment over several meetings. The advantage is that this creates an expectation that every session will be fifty minutes long. The disadvantage is that you may not get to the work of therapy for two or three weeks, and the client will become used to the idea of therapy as a series of question-and-answer sessions with very little hard work between them.

My own preference is to book the client for a longer assessment session (up to eighty minutes; an hour and a half slot in my schedule) and get through as much as possible in that first meeting. I let clients know this meeting will be longer than usual so they don't feel cheated when subsequent sessions end after fifty minutes. If I need to carry out more assessment tasks in subsequent sessions, I intermingle them with therapeutic tasks. My mission is to get to work as soon as possible, and by the end of the first session, I always know enough to be able to get started on something by the second meeting.

If you do this, should you charge for the extra time? I generally do not. If you choose to charge for a session and a half, be sure to let the client know beforehand. You do not want to surprise the client with a bill that is larger than expected.

ONE DAY A MONTH WITHOUT CLIENTS

You can always count on the odd slow day. Several clients have the flu, no one wants to come in on a certain day, or your biweekly folks have all bunched up on the same week, leaving alternate weeks with lots of gaps. On a slow day you can pick a project (transferring files from active to inactive storage, figuring out a tax issue, planning a talk) and get a lot of work done.

If your practice is reliably busy, however, you may find that you fall farther and farther behind on certain tasks, such as reports for insurers or thank-you notes to your referral sources. It's pleasant to schedule a monthly in-office vacation: a day in which you book no clients at all. You wear your jeans to work, settle in with your morning cup of coffee, turn on the radio, and lay out a limited number of tasks for the day.

These days can be incredibly productive. You don't have to clean up projects for incoming clients and, after they've left, refocus and figure out where you left off. You can spread paper all over the office to try to get an overview of what's happening. You can engage in messy tasks, such as shifting file cabinets around or cleaning up your bookcases and tossing out old journals. While doing this, avoid distractions: don't rush to answer the phone every time it rings and don't check your e-mail any more than usual. Imagine that the task before you is a living, breathing client, someone you would not interrupt for the phone or other distractions.

WATCH YOUR CLIENT LOAD

When setting your client load, draw a distinction between the number of clients you seem able to see in a single week and how many you can see week after week, year after year. These are two completely different numbers. If you overload yourself, you will eventually have to cut back sharply in order to regenerate. From month to month you will veer wildly from overload to underload, feeling stressed by the emotional drain on the high end and by the prospect of financial ruin on the low end. Instead, aim to see between half and three quarters of the number of clients you think you could handle if you were contemplating doing it only for one week.

Be sure you base your estimate on your mental and emotional capacity, not your financial goals or needs. If you see more clients than you can realistically manage, you will burn out anyway, and those goals will remain unmet. If your realistic capacity will bring in less money than you would like to make, you may need to think about adding another revenue stream: teaching a course at the university, taking a one-day-per-week job at a local hospital or agency, or doing time in a completely unrelated line of work. If the pay isn't as good as for clinical work, this is fine because additional clinical work above your realistic capacity is not a long-term option anyway.

Over time your capacity may shift. As you become more familiar with your client group, you may need less time between sessions to research, think, and plan. With practice and attention, your emotional boundaries may improve, allowing you to see highly distressed people without taking on their emotional burden.

Alternatively, you may tire of carrying a heavy clinical load. As you grow older, you may become increasingly aware that life is finite and that there is much you have not yet experienced. You may want more time for traveling, reading, or even hanging out on the beach. Perhaps you have a book to write, a cottage to build, or a university program you want to attend. Your energy may fade, making you just as, or even more, effective with the clients you see, but able to see fewer clients in a day or week. Shift your client load over time, rather than regard it as fixed.

USE AN ADVANCE PACKAGE

In private practice, clients (or insurers) pay for every moment the client sees you. It's important to make the most of that time. At intake we want to get the information we need from clients as efficiently as possible so we can deliver the service for which the client is actually seeing us.

Much of this information can be collected without the therapist's presence. You can ask clients to come in for thirty to sixty minutes before the first appointment to fill in some measures, or you can send an advance package to their homes for them to complete before their first appointment.

If you book assessment clients to come early to complete forms:

- You save the cost of postage.

- The forms won't be lost.

- The client won't forget to bring them in.

Managing Clinical Services

- You can ask the client to complete psychometrics that would be inappropriate to send in the mail.

- You or your assistant can answer any questions clients have while filling out the forms.

If, on the other hand, you send an advance package to clients' homes:

- You don't have to guess how long it will take clients to complete the forms.

- You can schedule clients' assessment appointments for first thing in the morning and you don't have to get there early.

- You can include a reminder appointment card.

- You can enclose an information sheet with the location of your building, how to get there, and where to park.

- You can include information on arranging payment through insurers.

- The client has longer to contemplate difficult questions: "What are your goals for therapy?" "Describe in your own words the difficulty you face."

- Clients have time to check on information they don't carry with them, such as their physicians' telephone numbers, the names of their medications, or the insurance reimbursement limit of their health plans.

On balance, many practitioners prefer to send an advance package. Of course, this isn't always possible. Sometimes clients don't want packages from therapists sent to their homes. Sometimes clients are booked with insufficient time for the mail to get to them. In these circumstances you can ask the client to come in early. Note that having clients come early is better than asking them to stay late. Some of the information will aid the first appointment, and some clients are so exhausted by the end of the assessment that they don't want to stay any longer.

Even if you mail an advance package, it's useful to ask new clients to come fifteen minutes early. At the first appointment clients probably won't know exactly where your office is, how long it takes to get there, where to park, and so on. They are more likely to be late for the assessment session than for any other appointment. Asking them to attend early maximizes the likelihood that they will be there when the appointment actually begins. If clients run a bit late, they won't have missed out on any of their time with you. If they get there on time, you will want to make sure the interval is spent well. You can ask clients to complete any measures you feel uncomfortable mailing out, and you or your assistant can look at what they have completed and score their questionnaires. That way you have some idea of what you're getting into when you invite the client into your office.

Of course, clients should be told when you will not be meeting with them right away and when the appointment may run long: "Most meetings here at the clinic are fifty minutes long, but please set aside an hour and a half to two hours for your first appointment. When you first arrive at the clinic, we will have a bit of administrative work to do, and then you will meet with Dr. Boring for an hour or perhaps a bit longer. So it's best not to schedule anything pressing for too soon after your appointment. Would that be all right?"

DEFINE THE PURPOSE OF THE INTAKE

Whenever you do anything, your chances of success are enhanced if you know what you are attempting to accomplish. Why are you assessing this person?

During your training, you could afford to spend a lot of time and be overinclusive, getting a full picture of the client's life, difficulties, personality, and history. In private practice your services are not free, and you cannot waste all of a client's resources or insurance coverage gathering reams of information. In some ways, most therapists' assessment training does them a disservice by failing to teach brevity and efficiency.

So why are you doing *this* assessment *now*? Maybe the purpose is to develop a session-by-session plan for therapy from start to finish. Though a nice idea, this approach presumes you will learn nothing more from the person once the intake is complete, which is unlikely and, in a sense, pessimistic. You will continue to have new insights about all clients all the way through your contact with them, and you will want to fine-tune your initial trajectory accordingly (hopefully without getting completely sidetracked).

So during the initial assessment process, you need to identify what you really need to know. Some of the factors involved are:

- The assessment question asked by your referral source

- The information you need to report to an insurer to secure coverage for subsequent sessions

- Information needed to create an initial case formulation and map out the first step or two of therapy

- The diagnosis, if this is likely to inform treatment selection

- The factors causing, supporting, and maintaining the presenting problem

- The compensatory strengths and coping strategies that have prevented the problem from being worse than it is or that have held off the problem until this point in the client's life

- Any imminent risks that need to be assessed or dealt with immediately

- Clients' reasons for coming to see you and their existing understanding of the problem and the means to its resolution

Perhaps there are other factors guiding the assessment for the type of clients you see. It would be worth taking some time with paper and pen to write them down. If you don't, you run the risk of being guided by the obsolete demands of the student role, or the functions of assessment at the job you had before starting private practice. For most private practitioners who assess for the purpose of guiding therapy, initial intake sessions are designed to fill in the rough outlines of a client's difficulty, with the understanding that additional information will appear as therapy progresses. Attempting to impose an illusory clarity from the outset may only straitjacket the process.

DEFINE THE FINISH LINE

How will you know when you are done? Therapy is like a good car: it can take you any number of places, but if you really want to get somewhere, it's best to have some idea of where you want to go. Both client and clinician should be clear on at least the rough outlines of the destination. If you do not do this, you run the risk of having your work with the client be governed by an irrational belief: *We'll stop meeting once the client has no problems left.* This, of course, will never happen, and therapy will end when you or the client finally gives up the quest. Work with the client to define the finish line, or else you may both drive off in the wrong direction.

Behavioral goals are the easiest to measure: "Get through my residency exam." "Go two months without visiting a casino." "Socialize with friends twice or more each week." Clients may want to specify cognitive or emotional goals, but even these can be made measurable: "A Beck Depression Inventory score below 15." "Fewer than two panic attacks a month." "Having a clear thing to say to myself when I become self-critical."

Sometimes this work reveals that the client has an exaggerated or inappropriate vision of what therapy can offer: "I never want to experience anxiety again." "I'll get up every morning looking forward to going to work." So long as the client holds unrealistic expectations, you are moving inexorably toward disappointment. Knowing that the client wants too much, you can address the issue of what to realistically expect before you get started.

Some clients are genuinely unclear about their goals. They don't know what kind of career would suit them. They're not sure whether to stay in their marriage or seek a divorce. This is the first task of therapy: exploring and defining the concept of the better life. If clarity is a problem, clarity becomes one of the goals.

PLAN SESSIONS IN ADVANCE

The financial side of private practice imposes an obligation to make the most of each session. If you wait until clients get in the room and see what comes up, you will almost certainly be conducting problem-of-the-week therapy: a recipe for ineffectiveness. Each week clients will come in with a different concern, which you will help them work on in a half-baked fashion; they will go away feeling vaguely better; and next week something else will come up. Eventually you will discover that none of the problems were fully dealt with, and your clients will be angry with you for wasting their time and money.

Instead, take part of the interval between clients to look at the notes and refresh your memory about the overall goals of therapy, the events of the previous session, the issues you need to follow up on, and the likely next steps you have identified. Consider making a few notes on your pad as reminders of the things you want to do. A list for one of my clients might look like this:

- Goals
- Dia br fu
- Cog intro
- Mother?
- Ins consent

"Goals" means I want to review the client's goals from last week and work with him to set new ones. "Dia br fu" means that in the last session I trained the client in diaphragmatic breathing, and now I should follow up ("fu") on it. "Cog intro" means it's time to introduce the basic cognitive model. "Mother?" might mean I know little thus far about the client's relationship with his mother, and I'd better ask. "Ins consent" means I need a release of information form signed so I can talk with the client's insurance case manager.

In effect, every session with a client is a meeting. You already know that meetings tend to be more productive with an agenda, so take the time to develop one and review it with the client at the outset of each session. Invite the client to add to the list. Avoid having so many items that the session is a sprint through the agenda; you will want time to process the new and unexpected. But avoid passively wandering through your meetings when time is limited and the expense is great.

PREPARE THE CONTAINER EVERY HOUR

A former colleague of mine had an office that can be described only as a nightmare. Stacks of paper sat on every horizontal surface, including on the floor and atop every bookcase. He insisted he knew where everything was and the just-ransacked-by-the-CIA look was an illusion. But anyone visiting him was overcome by a sense of barely restrained chaos. He seemed completely at ease in this environment. No one else did.

Clients arrive with a bundle of problems, symptoms, challenges, demands, and relationships that can feel hopelessly tangled. A great deal of therapy is about gently disentangling the threads of their lives, a calm sorting and processing of experience. Clients typically hope to achieve the peaceful calm of a still mountain lake. It is difficult to help clients reach this goal if the place where they work on it is not itself calm, peaceful, comfortable, and orderly. Consequently, each time we meet with a client, we should take a few moments to prepare the space. Here are the elements to consider:

- *Temperature:* If clients are either too warm or too cool, they will be distracted from the work. Considering and, if necessary, adjusting the heating before each appointment will avoid the distraction of having to open a window or fiddle with the thermostat during sessions.

- *Lighting and blinds:* As the sun moves and the weather changes, the lighting and mood in your office shift. Some times of day, either you or your client may be blinded; at other times your office will fall into cave-like darkness. Take a moment before each session to consider the position of your blinds and the level of the room lighting. If your office is visible from the street or from the building next door, you might choose always to have the blinds nearest the client tilted to enhance the sense of privacy. Most therapists will also want to avoid harsh fluorescent lights: too blue, too bright, and too clinical.

- *Seating:* Adjust the position of the chairs in the room, placing them at a comfortable distance from one another. If needed, adjust the location of the obligatory empty chair, and brush any crumbs, hairs, or other distractions from the client's chair.

- *Desk:* Clear the coffee table of paper and all clutter, and organize or put away the papers on your desk. The client wants to know that you have your life moderately together, and a desk in chaos belies this idea. It also makes clients wonder how carefully you maintain their files and information. A desk or credenza with multiple unfinished projects on it may also communicate that you are in the middle of something and might not really have time to sit and listen with your full attention.

- *No visible names:* Clients should never see documents or pieces of paper with other clients' names on them, or words they might believe to be someone's name. Even if the message is from your dentist, your client doesn't know that. You are aiming not only for complete confidentiality, but for the appearance of confidentiality as well.

- *Client's file face down:* In the course of an appointment, you may need to check something in a client's file, so you might want to have it on your desk ready for use. Place it face down so that the name is not visible. The client knows what it is, and you know what it is, so what does it matter? You don't want clients' eyes constantly drawn to their names on their files, distracting them with thoughts about what might be written inside. An even better procedure might be to have the client's file placed, alone, in the top drawer of your desk when the client comes in.

- *Clean whiteboard, pens ready:* If you have a whiteboard or flip chart, you'll want it clean and ready to use. Anything written on it will distract the client, who may wonder if it concerns another client (and if her own notes will be left for the next person to see). Whiteboards tend to get messy looking if frequently used; once a week consider cleaning it more thoroughly with spray.

Overall the principle is that there is typically enough disorder and confusion in people's minds as it is. The therapy space should be orderly, calm, and soothing, without a lot of distractions.

DEAL WITH PAYMENT AND BOOKINGS FIRST

Let's leap ahead for a moment. The session is almost over. You glance at the clock and see that you have a minute or two left. Another client is scheduled for the top of the hour. It's time to arrange the next meeting and deal with payment issues. What happens?

Usually everything is quick and smooth, but sometimes these chores take longer than expected. The client isn't available at the regular time next week, and you embark on a long exchange trying to find a good slot. The client rummages for the checkbook, stops to chat or ask questions between filling in each line of the check, then carefully records the check in the record book. The process often opens up new questions and topics: "How many more sessions do you think I should have?" "I'll be on vacation in October; would it be possible to have two sessions the week before I leave?" "My insurance company can now do direct billing; here's the form that sets it up."

All of these are perfectly legitimate topics for the client to want to cover, but now you're taking longer than expected and your note-writing time is evaporating. You'll be lucky to get to the next person on time even if you put off the note until later. You're beginning to experience a sense of time urgency that can look (or feel) like irritation if you're not careful. The longer the client takes, the more time he spends with you, so there is little incentive to hurry. You would have felt you were cheating the client if you'd started this whole process ten minutes before the session ended, so what can you do?

If you cannot off-load bookings and payments onto your assistant, then deal with them at the top of the session. The client comes in and sits down, and you have a receipt and your appointment book at the ready. For efficiency's sake, you book the next several appointments at once and verify the client's availability for all booked appointments at every session. You get the paperwork out of the way and then begin the session.

Isn't this cheating? Doesn't this just off-load this time into the client's valuable session time? Actually, no. Clients quickly learn that this is your routine, and they begin getting their payments ready and checking their schedules in the waiting room. They come into your room and hand you the payment already made out, and they're ready to set future meeting times. These two chores wind up taking at least 50 percent less time at the beginning than at the end of the session. Far from inconveniencing clients, you are giving them more useful therapy time. As well, you can use the recency effect to ensure that the last (and therefore most memorable) thing you say to the client has something to do with therapy, not paperwork.

PRACTICE THE TEN-MINUTE RULE

Everything takes time: telling a story, shifting to a new topic, coping with emotional content, introducing a new skill. Sometimes you can predict how long something will take; sometimes you can't. Avoid starting something you can't finish without running over time. As the session nears its end, begin using the time limitation as one consideration in your responses and interventions. The ten-minute rule is a useful (though not inviolate) touchstone: avoid magnifying emotion or switching to a new topic with less than ten minutes remaining in a session.

Let's say a client is telling you about a relative who made an unreasonable request, and you can see that the unexpressed reaction was a feeling of insignificance. Normally you might reflect the client's reaction to help him clarify and explore the issue, but history has taught you that this particular client is likely to become overwhelmed by his feelings. There may be tears, an outpouring of thoughts and interpretations, and an escalation into anger that will take time to subside. It's not so bad for a client to have an emotional experience toward the end of a session, but you don't want to strike a deep well of feeling and then spend the next five minutes pulling the client back, with your eye obviously on the clock.

It's useful, then, to think carefully before magnifying emotional material near the end of a session. Will this produce a productive insight, or will it lead to an awkward and ineffective end to your meeting, making it more difficult to cover the same ground in the future? "I'm noticing that this event really had a deep impact on you that might be very useful for us to explore. But I also want to give it the time it deserves, and we don't have that time just now. Would you be willing to revisit this next week?"

Similarly, if you know your diaphragmatic breathing lesson takes between ten and twenty minutes, avoid getting started on it with less than twenty minutes remaining. If your agenda has several topics left, consider switching to the one you can certainly cover in the time available. If the client placed something on the agenda and you don't have time to do it justice, ask permission to shelve it for the next appointment, at which time you will cover it early in the session. Alternatively, if you have an item that would fit nicely in the remaining time, point it out: "We've got a bit of time left, and I know you wanted to talk about your medication problem. Would now be a good time for that?"

It is the clinician's job to maintain the therapy space and to provide most of the structure in the work. The client should feel free to explore thoughts and feelings without the distraction of having to worry too much about timing issues. Some clinicians disagree, finding it too mechanistic or paternalistic to serve as timekeeper. The outcome, though, is often that the client loses track of time, opens a topic near the end, and is rudely awakened by the therapist's saying, "I'm afraid our time has run out for today." Regardless of your bias, it is best not to encourage the client to open topics that cannot be dealt with properly in the time available.

WRITE THE NOTES

In the course of a clinical day, you might find yourself pressed for time. The one thing you can always put off for later is writing session notes. At the end of a long day, you can find the temptation to head home almost overwhelming: "I'll do them tomorrow."

The longer you wait, and the more clients you see between the end of a session and the writing of notes, the more difficulty you will have when you get around to it. You may forget important details, neglect to record everything you did, and lose the sense you had of the logical next step in the work at session's end. It will also take you longer. The main function of your clinical notes (apart from legal or ethical requirements) is to jog your memory and help you to plan the work. You only make life more difficult for yourself when you put off writing your notes.

Consequently, it is best to force yourself to write notes at the end of every session, before seeing anyone else. If a delay is unavoidable, then write them as soon as possible—before heading out on your next break, for example. At minimum, ensure that all of your session notes are done before leaving for the day. Assessment reports, letters to lawyers or third-party insurers, billing notes, and e-mail replies can all wait. The completion of session notes, however, should be considered the requirement for an exit visa from the office. Every afternoon, you will regret establishing such a policy, but when you arrive each morning, you will be extremely glad you have it.

There you have it: a set of ideas for handling clients without imposing a specific therapeutic model or a batch of interventions. Practice these principles, and you will find that your clinical work proceeds much more smoothly than it would otherwise.

CHAPTER 10

The Ritual Clinic: Keeping Your Work Sustainable

Rituals are an essential aspect of every society. Indeed, to a great extent the nature of these rituals defines the culture: how we wash, eat, play, socialize, mate. Ritual has a bad name in many Western circles because it is taken to be a meaningless constraint on freedom, but ritual is universal because it works. Ritual is structure: a skeleton that the meat of our lives is built around.

We all have personal rituals, or habits, as well: coffee before newspaper, pizza night on Thursdays. They simplify life, reduce the weight of decision making ("Should I shower first or brush my teeth first?"), and leave our minds free to focus on what matters. The importance of our rituals intrudes on our consciousness only when they are disrupted. In our clients' lives, the breakdown of structure and ritual (going to work, getting out of bed at the same time each day, dressing in clean clothes) can signal the worsening of a disorder, and part of the task of therapy can be to help them rebuild structure into their lives.

Private practice removes much of the structure imposed by the needs, policies, and whims of a large organization. For many clinicians, the freedom from meaningless routine is one of the main attractions of working for yourself. But structure, routine, and ritual are necessary to prevent life from becoming overwhelming. Many practices fail because clinicians neglect to put new rituals in place that will sustain the business—and the clinician's stability.

The question is not whether ritual will form a part of your work life. The question is whether you will consciously choose your rituals or whether they will simply accumulate like barnacles on a ship's hull.

Much of this book has been about developing the rituals of a successful practice. In this chapter, we consider habits not for the creation of a new practice, but for the longevity and stability of the clinician. The intent is not to impose a Stalinist regime of rigid structure bounded by walls of concrete and barbed wire. Instead, we want personalized guidelines, freely chosen, that will enhance our sense of satisfaction and freedom, alleviating the necessity to reorganize every day, rethink every task, and devote scarce mental resources to problems for which solutions have already been found.

ARRIVE AT WORK BEFORE YOU WORK

One morning I opened my office door, crossed to the telephone, tapped in the voice-mail code, and began writing down messages before my coat was off. I realized I had been doing this for weeks and was starting each day in a state of mild agitation as a result. I created a new rule: when I arrived at the office, I would hang up my coat, sit down, and breathe for a minute or two before doing anything else. This proved to be a useful way of helping me prepare for the day ahead.

The demands of work differ from the rest of your life, and you assume a completely different role as you cross the threshold of your office. Physically you may have arrived, but it takes time for your mind to adjust. Recognize this, acknowledge it, and give yourself time to assume the mantle of the clinician. Here are some of the transition strategies reported by clinicians in my informal survey:

- Walk the dog as the last thing before leaving for work.

- Walk to work, formulating a mental list of priorities for the day.

- Walk to work, deliberately setting aside thoughts of the office until arriving there.

- Listen to music en route to avoid obsessing about the practice.

- Go directly from parking lot to coffee shop to sit and contemplate the day ahead.

- Arrive at work and do several minutes of meditation (or yoga) before doing anything else.

Whatever the circumstances of your own practice, make a point of punctuating the transition from home to work with something calming and orienting. Ritualize the transition so that you begin to do it automatically, without having to think about it (a "Home-to-Work Transition" worksheet is available at the websites noted in the introduction). Don't ignore this task if you have a home office. Instead, take even more time to think it through. Clinical work is a different way of thinking, a different way of being. It takes effort to put your everyday concerns away so that they don't play out with clients, and to orient your mind to the role of helper, observer, coinvestigator, and coach.

EAT THE FROG

There are dozens, perhaps hundreds, of chores involved in running a practice. Most days you will be faced with a list of them, some appealing and others less so. Which should you do first?

One time-honored strategy is to put everything off long enough that something becomes a crisis, thus imparting enough adrenaline-fueled motivation that you can accomplish it. Another is to do whatever appeals to you the most at the moment. These strategies leave unpleasant but necessary tasks undone for extended periods of time. This is problematic because tasks can take up mental space in two ways: the time spent getting them done, and the time spent berating yourself for not having done them before now. Unpleasant chores keep emerging from the papers on your desk, bludgeoning you with your failure and lack of discipline before they are hastily reshuffled to the bottom of the pile.

Nicolas de Chamfort (1741-1794) once said, "A man should swallow a toad every morning to be sure of not meeting with anything more revolting in the day ahead." Time management guru Brian Tracy (2001) has adapted this idea as one of his many strategies for increasing work efficiency. He suggests that each morning there are dozens of tasks on your desk needing to be "eaten," and among them is an enormous, slimy, unappetizing frog. That frog, or de Chamfort's toad, will sit staring at you all day, spoiling the enjoyment you get from doing anything else until it is finally ingested.

The suggestion, then, is to look at your to-do list and find the one item that gives you the strongest feeling of reluctance and repulsion—the most powerful temptation to set it aside. Do that task first. The result will be a sensation of lightness and momentum. Everything else on your list will look trivial by comparison. Having disposed of your frog, the day already feels like a success even if you accomplish nothing else. Crises will develop less often, and you will have much less cause to berate your lack of discipline.

LIMIT MAIL CHECKING

Earlier I advocated checking your voice mail (or having someone else check it) several times a day, given that new referrals tend to have a short half-life. There is a limit to this policy, however. Your e-mail and voice mail can be very much like slot machines: every so often they pay off with something interesting: a new referral, a request to deliver a talk, a note from a friend. Intermittent reinforcement is, as we know, the most effective way to encourage a high rate of behavior, and this is exactly what our voice mail and e-mail accounts provide. Many professionals feel an almost irresistible compulsion to check both at every opportunity. This is both unproductive and anxiety inducing.

It takes perhaps a few seconds to download new e-mails, but it takes longer to check what you have received, delete spam, and decipher the contents of the rest. Meanwhile, you have diverted your attention from what you were doing. It takes several minutes to refocus when you are done. The more frequently you check, the more often you expend this effort for nothing. As well, most people become more efficient when they respond to multiple e-mails at one time, making quick decisions and rattling off replies. When you check every hour, you lose this advantage.

I recommend checking e-mail and voice mail early in the day, before your first session. (It may, after all, let you know that your first client has the flu and can't make the appointment.) Then leave both for an hour or two, and check again at a midmorning break or just before lunch. Then check again at midafternoon and before leaving for home. Leave it alone at other times. Most of the perceived urgency in messages is illusory. As well, replying to e-mails instantly encourages people to rely on your rapid responses. They will write you with questions rather than think for themselves, send you a flurry of e-mails rather than a single one, and reply to you with their next messages more quickly. One way to reduce the number of e-mails you get is to reply only a day or two after receiving them.

IF YOU WANT IT TO HAPPEN, WRITE IT DOWN

A paper or electronic daybook is standard equipment for any clinician. For the past fifteen years, I have used a page-per-day appointment book. One year I experimented with an electronic system but found that it took me longer to record appointments, it was hard to see what my entire week looked like, it was easy to make mistakes (like scheduling clients for 10:00 p.m. instead of 10:00 a.m., resulting in double bookings), and I couldn't bother using it to write extended notes (such as the agenda for a meeting or the directions to a workshop site). Eventually I gave up and returned to my daybook. When you drop a daybook on the floor, all the appointments are still in it when you pick it up.

Whether you use paper or electrons, what should go into your daybook? Your client appointments, obviously, plus other scheduled commitments: committee meetings, supervision sessions, teleconferences, continuing-education events, tax deadlines, dental appointments, dinner dates, and concerts. At one point in your life, you may have been able to keep track of your life in your head. If that time was not well and truly past when you started your private practice, it will be soon, so stop relying on it.

What about all of the things you have to do that are not clearly tied to a certain time? Report writing, shopping for supplies, sending thank-you notes, setting up new computers, reading the literature, performing a thousand clinic-management tasks—how can you be sure that you won't forget them and that they will actually get done?

One option is to use an additional list-making application for your computer or smartphone. Being a Luddite (apparently), I solve this problem by using a small lined notebook. At the start of a week, I create new pages for business and personal chores that need completing ("Apr 20–24—Work" and "—Pers") and write down items as I think of them. Because the book is small enough to carry with me wherever I go, I can write down tasks as I think of them, and I don't have to rely on memory. Anything that isn't tied to a specific week (book ideas, holiday plans, talks I want to give someday, yearly goals, and so on) gets entered on pages at the back of the book. When the filled pages in front and back meet in the middle (which takes me about a year), it's time for a new notebook. I could easily use a similar system with lined pages in my daybook, but I like the portability of a smaller book.

What if you have something you keep meaning to do, but it never seems to happen? Schedule it on your calendar the way you would any meeting. If you do this, get in the habit of treating these appointments as seriously as your client sessions. Don't let them slide ("That's just a note to myself; I can do that anytime"). Treat the ritual seriously if you want it to be valuable. If you're not sure you're going to honor an appointment with yourself, don't write it down. When your time to "Complete Smith report" comes around, set other things aside and do it. Never book the whole day this way, however, because you need uncommitted time to respond to crises, goof off, take longer phone calls, and so on. If there isn't any unstructured time in a day, you will get in the habit of robbing your self-appointments for it, and their value will be lost.

PLAY AT WORK

One option for your private practice is to keep work and leisure clearly separate. Another is to introduce a bit of fun and levity into the workplace. When asked how they avoid burnout, several of my colleagues stated that they deliberately incorporate leisure and "nonwork" into each day, which helps them to decompress from what can be emotionally draining work. A bit of levity and leisure can act like a sorbet between courses at a formal dinner. It cleanses the palate, setting aside the leftover "taste" from the preceding session and opening your receptivity for what is to come.

We become so accustomed to our grade-school teachers' admonishment to "stop playing around" that we can feel a vague sense of guilt when a supervisor at work passes in the hallway as we describe our vacation plans to a coworker. It is built into our automatic thinking that at work we should be working and anything else is a distraction. In private practice the boss has been vanquished, but her ghostly presence (a half-sensed projection of your own superego) remains. As well, we get paid only when we produce, so there is a temptation to put aside all trivial and childish things and focus exclusively on the work. But the work may suffer as a result.

It can be a good idea to confront the ghost directly and announce that you have every intention of enjoying your time at work. You are an adult, after all, and it is *your* work, *your* practice, and *your* life. Furthermore, your work will be more effective if it is not soulless and driven, like that of a seamstress in an industrial-revolution sweatshop. You will be a better clinician if you have a little sorbet now and then.

So make a point of conversing with the other people in the office. Hang about in the waiting room. Chat about your weekend. Book tickets to an upcoming concert. Bring in a trashy novel to read during your breaks. Be inefficient and irresponsible for at least part of every day.

Notice a disconnect that you would be quick to point out to clients. There are pastimes that are tempting to contemplate and ones that are satisfying to *do*. If you do not give your play the serious attention it deserves, you will fall into the trap of amusing yourself with obsessive and fundamentally unsatisfying activities: randomly surfing the Internet, reading and rereading the news, playing game after game of computer solitaire. Expunge unsatisfying obsessions from your day and replace them with activities you actually enjoy doing.

GET OUT OF THE OFFICE

With severely depressed clients, one of the tasks is to help them reintroduce structure into their lives. One of the most useful guiding principles is the idea that every day, they should get out of the house at least once, even if it is just to the corner store or to pull one weed out of a flower bed.

What's good for our clients is usually good for us as well. The life of a therapist is excessively sedentary, and it can be tempting to sit in the office all day with the walls slowly closing in on us. So make a point of leaving the office at least once a day.

The most obvious recommendation is to go out for lunch. Don't simply fetch it back to your desk. Make dates with your office colleagues, if you have some. Take your assistant to lunch at least once a month—and make sure you pick up the tab. Survey the neighborhood for friends who work nearby. Push past your inertia and call them up to book lunches with them.

Here are some other options: A midday workout can split up your client load, reenergize you, and give you a much-needed lift to get you past the early-afternoon slump. You can also retain some tasks you might otherwise pass off to your assistant: getting the mail, buying stationery supplies, running to the printer. Become the tea wallah for the office, supplying your colleagues and assistant with their morning caffeine and afternoon decaf.

MARK THE TRANSITION FROM WORK TO HOME

Conducting therapy is not like cutting lumber, stocking shelves, or selling handbags: easy to leave behind you and impossible to do much about in your off-hours. You can think about your clients endlessly, and their challenges can follow you into your private life. When you have a private practice, business details can come home with you as well. Are you making enough money? Did you remember to submit the quarterly payroll statement? Should you send out more pamphlets? When your workday is filled with conceptual material as potent as the work of therapy and business, it becomes important to mark the transition from work to home—to ritualize the shift so that your mind makes it a habit to let go of work and allow you to be present at home. (A "Work-to-Home Transition" worksheet is available at the websites noted in the introduction.)

Different therapists have different rituals. The walk home, if you are fortunate enough to live close to your office, is ideal. But do not rely on the walk itself; it's easy to obsess about work issues until you are suddenly confronted by your arrival at your front door. Gently bring your mind into the present: the tree that's showing signs of coming into leaf, the changing posters at the video store, the distinct shape of the clouds. Even reviewing your plans for the evening can orient you toward home rather than work.

One therapist in my survey reported that when she drives into her parking space at home she makes a point of sitting there, breathing, for a full three minutes before getting out of the car. Her children, dog, and husband instantly compete for her attention when she opens the front door, so she needs a bit of time alone first. Another clinician reported that she changes her clothes the moment she arrives home, taking off her work role along with the professional uniform. Another makes a point of washing her face. Several reported that they immediately take the dog for a walk, out of necessity as well as ritual. Others get on the carpet and play with the cat.

In your work you talk with people all day long about their issues. Your partner, if you have one, may not have quite so social a job. If your partner stays home to care for the kids or work from a home office, he is probably starved for contact with an adult—*any* adult, not just you. Consequently, whereas you may need some quiet time during which you don't have to talk or think about anyone else's needs, your partner may long for discussion and a review of the day. This is a potential source of frustration. One solution is the fifteen-minute rule, in which the person arriving home is ritually afforded fifteen minutes before having to listen to any stories about the day or answer any questions. The principle works both ways. Even if you are the type who likes to breeze into the house and launch into a soliloquy about your day, your partner may be so exhausted by work or the homeward commute that she cannot bear to speak for a time.

What about the rest of your social network? Lawyers attract legal questions. Physicians are asked to inspect suspicious moles. Therapists often get friends relating their own distressing issues—either because we are good listeners or because we are so tired of talking all day that we sit staring, apparently attentive, when someone unpacks his traumas in our vicinity. Sometimes we learn from our home e-mail or voice mail that a friend would really like to come over for a chat and a glass of wine or simply wants us to call back. Doing the mental arithmetic, we realize it's about time for that friend's divorce agreement to arrive in the mail, another disagreement with the person's brother, or a problem with a child. We are compassionate people, and it can feel like—and be—a great privilege to be our friends' trusted confidante. But perhaps a part of your ritual must be to put off the return call until you have had dinner and some time to decompress.

COLLEGIAL CONTACT

One of the major drawbacks of private practice is the potential for isolation. When you work for a hospital, a prison system, or a mental health center, though you may have to put up with a great deal of administrative nonsense, you have the benefit of colleagues with whom you can consult, go to lunch, or complain. Some private practices have many clinicians, but most are small operations where consulting with colleagues can be a challenge.

There are various results of isolation. Loneliness is an obvious one: if every day you go to work, unlock the door to your small suite, do a bit of paperwork while awaiting the first client, see a stream of people with whom you are not entitled to share your life and problems, and then lock up and head home, you may feel that you live in a kind of alternate universe of sadness and trauma. A sense of insignificance is another result: you toil away, attempting to banish depression, anxiety, or psychosis, feeling that you are trying to empty an ocean of mental distress with a teaspoon. An excess of confidence is a less obvious, but no less significant, problem: you inch beyond standard practice, gradually shifting your techniques and believing in what you do until your treatment style is entirely idiosyncratic and contrary to the evidence.

It is essential to remain tethered to some semblance of professional reality through regular contact with your fellow clinicians. You can accomplish this task in a number of ways:

Do lunch. Set up a regular lunch date with a colleague who practices in your area of town. If it isn't regular (say, the third Wednesday of each month), you will quickly fall out of the habit. Talk about your practice, your career, and your challenging cases (the details heavily disguised, of course). Pick a restaurant where the tables are sufficiently spaced that you can feel comfortable in the discussion.

Get supervision. Set up regular consultation sessions with an experienced senior clinician or mentor. You might use these sessions to review your most difficult cases. Alternatively, if the person is more of a practice coach, you can use her to help guide your career and development.

Start or join a consultation group. Many communities have groups of clinicians who get together every month or two to discuss difficult clients and try out new intervention strategies. Some clinicians belong to reading groups or journal clubs, in which the members take turns choosing readings and leading discussions. If there are no such groups in your area, consider forming one.

Enter therapy. You probably tell clients that being in therapy is no sign of weakness but rather an indication of a resolve to produce helpful change. If you actually believe this, then why not try it yourself? It can be tempting to say that you have no issues to work on, but surely you are not subject to that level of delusion. Sitting on the other side of the tissue box can be tremendously enlightening about the experience your clients face in therapy. You can notice your own resistance to pressure, your response to metaphor, and the ebb and flow of your enthusiasm for the process as time passes and as your therapist shifts strategies. You need not enroll in decade-long psychoanalysis, but having the occasional session with a trusted and admired professional can help you to maintain perspective, preserve the balance in your life, and learn new ways of being with your own clients.

Have a mentor or coach. The difference between mentors and coaches is usually financial: mentors typically do it for enjoyment, while coaches do it as a career. Mentors can be hard to find; you have to discover them, they must really want to help, and they will usually serve as mentors to a very limited number of people. Coaches are easier to find but can be more difficult to evaluate. You will want to know a coach's training and area of particular expertise. You could search for a coach or consultant who could help you fine-tune your practice with certain client groups or with a specific model of therapy. Another option is a business coach, who could help you set goals and work toward creating a functioning private practice.

Whatever you decide, do not spend the rest of your professional life alone in an office seeing clients. It will become boring or overwhelming, and your much-sought-after freedom will become a curse.

ATTEND CONTINUING-EDUCATION EVENTS REGULARLY

Most regulated professions require that you participate in some kind of continuing education. Whether yours does or not, it is a very good idea to take part. Knowledge did not cease being gathered the day we graduated, and we have all met the senior practitioner who has apparently not learned a thing (nor read a book) for the past thirty years. Believing that we have mastered our field is narcissism, not insight.

Workshops, conferences, and seminars have other benefits as well. They can reengage us with our work, provide a different perspective on what we have been doing, and show us that others share our challenges. Workshops, with their intensive focus on one topic, can help us to grasp much of a new area. Conferences, which are like twenty-one-ring circuses, can be more motivational.

To make the most of these events, arrive early and make a point of mingling at breaks. Attend the social events and try not to hang out with the one or two people you already know, unless you make a point of introducing each other to new people. The breaks and after-hours periods of conferences (in particular) can be the most valuable part of the experience. If you have to travel to attend, consider taking an extra day or two to relax and sightsee.

TAKE VACATIONS REGULARLY

The working world is full of people who drop into casual conversation the fact that they seldom take vacations. Sometimes they reveal this with mock shame, thinly disguising their pride at being such dedicated employees, such responsible people, such hardworking citizens. They may clearly hate their work, making such dedication seem pointless, or they may be neglecting (or avoiding) their families, but there persists the sense that working without cease is a virtue.

Elsewhere in this book I have made the rather obvious point that private practice entails no paid vacation whatsoever. When you contemplate taking a week or two off, a part of your mind will tabulate the revenue you will forego and the overhead (such as rent) that will accrue anyway. So taking time off will cost you money—even before you pay for airfare, hotels, or any of your vacation expenses. The temptation, inevitably, will be to keep working. You can do this for a while, but eventually you will need time away to renew your motivation, as well as to reconnect with yourself and your life outside work.

Why do you want your business to be a success? Doubtless one goal is to contribute to your community and to the health and welfare of others. But even this can be in service to another goal that you almost certainly harbor, which is to be happy: *I'll be a respected professional and business owner, help others, make a good income, and feel fulfilled in my life.* Working ceaselessly will not bring you to this destination. You may make more money for a while (until you burn out), but you will probably not be happy. Time spent with family, with your friends, with your partner, or even in relaxed solitude often proves to be a much more efficient generator of happiness than overwork.

So take your vacations. Talk back to the voice that shouts about the cost of taking time off, and remind yourself of the cost of not doing so. One of the main goals of private practice is freedom, not enslavement. Be sure to take at least as many vacation days as you did when you last worked for someone else. But why stop there? It truly is your life and your career. You could take nine weeks each year if you want. I do.

When do you book time off? One strategy is to wait for the telltale signs of impending burnout. This is like waiting for angina before starting an exercise routine. Instead:

- Plan time off in advance so that you have something to look forward to. Vacations are beneficial in anticipation, as well as in practice. Having an upcoming holiday to contemplate is one of the pleasures of life, and it can help us through those moments when things get difficult: *Never mind, I'll soon be on the beach.*

- Take chunks large enough to truly decompress. The demands of clients can make it hard to contemplate taking more than a week at a time. Many people find, however, that it takes at least a week to slow down and for their minds to stop hunting for chores that need to be done. The true vacation begins when you let go of your life, and if this occurs only the day before the flight home, then the vacation is unlikely to satisfy. At least one or two vacations each year should be longer than a week.

- Have your next vacation planned before you return from the previous one. When you come home, you can feel let down at no longer having something to look forward to. So plan two vacations ahead. Even on that first day back, the next vacation will beckon. You might not know exactly where you are going or what you will do, but you know that three months from now, you will, again, take a break.

MAXIMIZE VACATION IMPACT

Vacations are meant to be restorative. A few tricks that ensure and enhance this effect include:

Avoid taking new clients before going on vacation. When clients have a first appointment, they often get charged up and ready to get to work on the problem. This surge of interest will tend to fade if they don't act on it within a few weeks. As well, your own recollection and understanding of the client may dissipate while you are on vacation. If departing clients leave you with gaps in your schedule, use the resulting free time to complete projects and get caught up on the clinic's day-to-day chores.

Avoid seeing clients late on your last day. It's tempting—and sometimes unavoidable—to overbook clients for the last few days before vacation. Avoid booking them for late afternoon on your final day, however. Invariably (judging from my own experience) your final client will be in crisis, and you will leave with a sense of incompletion or anxiety that will follow you onto the plane. Even if this doesn't happen, you will wind up stuck in your office, cleaning up and writing that last note later than you ordinarily would. Other crises may also tend to cluster on your final day. Colleagues, assistants, clients, and others often procrastinate before giving you unwelcome information, so it is often just before you head off for a few weeks that you learn that someone is quitting and needs a reference letter, that the computer is not working properly, that your assistant urgently needs to be paid but hasn't completed the time sheet, or that the funding on a project is in danger. If you leave that final afternoon clear of clients, you will almost certainly be glad you did.

Take client contact information on holiday with you. Flights get delayed. Trains derail. Highways wash out. Sooner or later you are going to be delayed while returning from a vacation. In a private practice no one may be able to cover for you. Take along a copy of your appointment schedule for your first couple of days back, plus the

The Ritual Clinic: Keeping Your Work Sustainable

telephone numbers of the clients you have booked (as well as your assistant's e-mail address and home phone number). Use initials or some other disguise so you don't have to worry quite so much about confidential information. If you are delayed, you can call people and cancel.

Clean your desk before going away. The last thing you do before heading out the door should be to organize your workspace. This will help you to let go of your practice, knowing that things are left in an orderly way with most loose ends resolved. More important, when you get back, you will open your office door and see the clean, calm surface of your desk rather than a chaotic jumble of papers you no longer recognize. The vacation effect will last longer.

Don't assume that relaxation will relax you. Some people fantasize about lying by a pool with a book but find that by the third day of such a vacation, they are hopelessly bored. Let's face it: sitting at your desk with a cup of tea is already physically relaxing; you may not need more inactivity. The most restorative vacations are often those that balance your regular routine with the opposite. A week of kayaking in Haida Gwaii will almost certainly do you more good than sipping forty-two piña coladas on a beach.

Plan what you want, not what vacation planners are selling. If you walk into the average travel agency, you might think absolutely everyone wants to be standing knee-deep in blue water in front of a concrete tower: *Oh, that's what a vacation looks like.* If you are one of the many who are not suited to wading, you might be tempted to conclude that vacations are not for you. Think back to the things you have really enjoyed. Perhaps you would like to attend a science fiction or hockey card convention, hike the backcountry, visit your old college friend Muriel in Cincinnati, or meditate for a month at a retreat center.

Vacation at home—but with caution. Now and then it can be refreshing to take vacation days in town. You can hang out with friends, make elaborate dinners, see movies and cultural events, take day trips, and visit the attractions tourists usually seek out. The problem is the siren song of the office. When you leave town on vacation, you can't drop into the clinic to see a client or fill out a tax form. At home you can, and your vacation will be much less of a break if you give in to the temptation. You can also do so many household chores that you feel just as worn out as at the end of a long workweek. If you want to vacation at home, then vacation. Do not permit yourself to "catch up" on your work or home projects. If you take a week off to focus on a household task, such as painting the house, then either do not count this as a vacation, or force yourself to take evenings and breaks to meet with friends and do all the other things you would do on a true vacation.

Alternate your types of vacation. It is possible to burn out on the same type of vacation, just as we can burn out working at the same type of job day after day. Create some variety in the breaks you take: mountains, beaches, home, great cities, cruises, adventure tours, volunteer work, retreat centers.

Limit contact with home. A break is restorative because it is a break, not because it enables you to keep your finger on the pulse of everything at work. E-mail, the Internet, cheap long-distance rates, and the ubiquity of cell phones allow us to stay in intimate contact with our lives no matter where we are. For a real break, immerse yourself in the vacation and sharply limit your connection with home. Check your e-mail and voice mail as seldom as you can, and make sure your assistant knows that his primary function while you are away is to serve as a buffer between you and work, handling or delaying as much as he possibly can and contacting you only if absolutely necessary.

Allow brainstorming. When you think about a problem intently and then set it aside and relax (as Archimedes did in his bathtub), ideas can suddenly pop into your head. When you take a break from work, you can get flashes of a larger perspective: *I've taught that extension course for the last three years. It pays just about nothing, and I'm bored.*

Maybe I'll give it up. I've been mentoring Anne about setting up her practice. What if I invited her to join mine? This can be one of the great benefits of vacations. So although it is a good idea to set most work aside, it's fine to carry a notebook and keep a record of the thoughts that pop up while you are traveling.

BOOK WORK AROUND YOUR LIFE, NOT YOUR LIFE AROUND WORK

One of the primary attractions of private practice is flexibility. A large organization will usually tell you when to arrive in the morning, what days to work, and when to go home, expecting you to organize your life around those boundaries. In private practice you get to decide. It is surprising how many clinicians automatically opt for a nine-to-five, Monday-to-Friday workweek in the absence of external constraints, as though it were somehow a law of the universe.

When building your practice, consider the particulars of your life. Imagine that there are no expectations, no norms dictating what a workweek looks like. If you have children, it is completely legitimate to build your schedule to suit child-care needs or your daughter's soccer games. If you like to travel, who says you can't take twelve weeks of vacations a year? If you like to work at home in your pajamas, why not schedule all of your client appointments on two or three days and stay at home the rest of the time? If you're a night owl, why would you ever work mornings?

Try to detect superego poisoning, which may tell you that your life, preferences, and needs are trivial and that you should feel guilty for making them a priority. To be sure, few clients will want to see you at 3:00 a.m., and perhaps it will be difficult to shunt your clinic days around randomly from week to week. But the balance between the demands of your practice and those of your life should be a negotiation, not a defeat. If your market is good enough and your needs few enough, you can do pretty much whatever you like.

In addition to building an overall picture of your work life to suit your needs, consider your day-to-day decisions. Clients will tell you they can't come in during regular work hours, they need to see someone on a Saturday, or they want an "approximate" appointment so they don't have to rush to get to your office at a specific time. You are the one offering the service. It is entirely legitimate to decide what you will and will not offer, and to stick to it. Perhaps you don't work late Tuesdays so you and your buddies can go bowling. This may seem trivial to you relative to the difficulties your clients face, and you may be tempted to give it up. You can do this now and then if you like, but you should keep in mind why you went into private practice. If the freedom to set your own work hours is important to you, think twice before changing things. The question is not whether you can survive if you give up bowling this once or if you come in to work despite feeling truly ill. It is whether you will continue to enjoy the work if you routinely make a practice of ignoring your life and your needs to suit your clients' wishes.

The same principle holds for your nonclinical work. A member of the professional association wants to know if you will serve on a committee. A faculty member at the local university has a student getting ready for her Ph.D. defense and wonders if you can serve as the external examiner. The head of the citizen's advocacy group wants to know if you will help out during mental health week. An old graduate-school buddy calls, asking if you will write a chapter for her upcoming book. They all sound interesting, but agreeing to everything will ultimately sink your enthusiasm for your practice if you are not careful. Your interest will cause you to agree to almost anything, and sooner or later you will be so overloaded your life will seem like a trial.

You need a brake on your enthusiasm, guilt, and overestimation of your own capacity for efficiency. Base your decisions not on whether you can cope this week or this month, but on whether you could cope if the decision you made and the load you took on lasted indefinitely. It can help to have a mantra to rely on. My colleague Martha Capreol reminded me of a useful one: "This is a marathon, not a sprint." Could you run faster? Yes. Could you run faster all the way to the finish line? No. Then don't speed up.

NEVER TAKE ON A PROJECT THE DAY IT IS OFFERED

As your career progresses, you will get asked to take part in dozens of projects, reports, research studies, planning sessions, committees, and boards. Inevitably you will find yourself overcommitted. The sign of this is obvious enough: a rising tide of anxiety, a feeling of being overwhelmed by all of the things you have to do. You begin to wonder whether you will ever be able to live up to people's expectations, given the number of obligations in your week.

That feeling and those thoughts are tremendously useful. They are signals that you have steered your course toward exhaustion. You can use them to set a new rule: *I'm not allowed to take on anything new this month.* Unfortunately, the next thing you are offered will be something that is perfectly suited to your interests and would be good for your practice.

Another option is not to wait for a complete overload before putting a hand on the wheel. You could ration yourself based on what you know about your capacity: *I'm allowed to sit on two committees, one board, and one research project. So I'd better be sure that anything I take on is something I really want to do.*

How do you ensure this? Never agree to a project on the day it is offered to you. Pledge that you will put off all requests for at least one day before signing on. To do this, you have to have a set of stock responses at the back of your mind, because you never know when people are going to ask you to do something. Develop your standard replies alone, then rehearse them (perhaps in front of the mirror) until they feel natural and you know them so well that you don't have to think hard to come up with them.

- "That sounds like a great idea. I'm going to have to check my schedule, and I'll e-mail you Tuesday."
- "Thank you for asking me. Do you have a card, and I'll get back to you tomorrow?"
- "I have a lot going on right now. Let's talk about it at the next meeting."

Needless to say, you also need a set of stock replies when you know immediately that a project is not for you.

- "Thank you so much for asking. I'm really trying to focus my efforts on just a few things right now, though, so I'm not adding new projects to the list."
- "That sounds like a great idea, and I hope it goes really well. I'm working on another research project at the moment, and I'm afraid there's only so much time in a day."
- "I've finally figured out that I am just not a committee person, so I don't sit on them anymore."

I realized about fifteen years ago that my reflexive answer to almost any request was yes. This sounds honorable, as though it reflects spontaneity and openness to new experiences. I hope that this is partly true, but I also know that I have a powerful desire to please people and an irrational fear that every opportunity is the last one I'll be offered. I eventually adopted the "tell you tomorrow" rule during a time when I was seriously overcommitted, and it gradually became second nature. It served me well, and I have kept it ever since.

In this chapter we have considered a number of strategies for managing a practice over the long term, with the goal of sustainability. There are other tricks, and perhaps you have discovered some

The Ritual Clinic: Keeping Your Work Sustainable

of them yourself. They constitute the lane markings on the highway of practice.

Although helpful, these techniques do not guarantee us against veering off the highway completely into the land of burnout. To reduce the likelihood of this common hazard to private practitioners, more is necessary. In the next chapter we will consider strategies for preventing burnout and recovering from it.

CHAPTER 11

The Long View: Burnout and Beyond

When I returned to Vancouver in the early 1990s after a long absence, a friend from graduate school had preceded me. Richard had opted to take up sailing, and I decided to take a class with him. Our lessons spread through that first winter. We would go out into English Bay in the driving rain. No other boats would be there. We threw floats overboard and practiced sailing off to a count of ten, whipping around, and retracing our course to pluck them out of the water, trying not to fall overboard ourselves. Sailing was a miserable business. Richard bought a sailboat. I did not.

The lessons were many years ago, but sailing metaphors still creep into my clinical work. One of them is that you sail with your mind in three places. You're focused on what you're doing, trying to do it properly while the deck pitches beneath you. You pay attention to the water just ahead, watching for rocks, floating debris, and other boats. If you're not careful, those two objects of focus will occupy you completely, and you will neglect the third: your destination. Where are you trying to go? In a tidal current you can aim straight for Point Atkinson and still miss it completely. Hopefully you know enough to take the current into account when plotting your course. Even then, however, you need to watch your progress, and correct and correct and correct again.

Operating a psychotherapy practice is similar. It is possible to get so caught up in the tasks of the moment that you fail to steer the business. Much of this book has been designed to help you decide where you would like your practice to go and how to work the rudder. The intent of this final chapter is to take the longer view, to survey the course ahead in terms of years rather than days or months.

If the real reasons we do most things are to contribute to the world and to be happy, then how can we contribute for the long haul? How can we be happy with the journey as well as the destination it takes us toward?

One of the critical issues here is burnout. Most therapists can get started and build a practice, whether on their own or as part of a larger organization. But few escape hints of burnout along the way. If getting through your career without even a whiff of burnout is an unrealistic goal (and it is), then how can you avoid letting it get the better of you? If you follow many of the recommendations in the preceding chapters, you will find that you miss many of the rocks that could puncture your hull. You will have a balanced client load, you will have less stress about income, you will be able to off-load duties to your assistant. In this chapter, let's point out a few more.

And what then? You may not want to run a practice forever. How can you arrange the transition to whatever comes next so that you do not destabilize your life completely? It is always more comfortable being in a room if you can see the exit. Even if you plan to carry on indefinitely, knowing how to get out can help. But before we talk about the distant future, let's consider some ways to help get you there.

LIVE THE LIFE YOU RECOMMEND

What do we suggest our clients do in order to feel better? Usually we have some specific recommendations based on the particular problem, but often our advice is quite generic. We conduct a careful appraisal of our clients' day-to-day existence and suggest strategies for shifting their routines toward a more healthy and sustainable life. These changes may not resolve deep-seated issues, but they can bring the client to a place of strength from which the real issues can be addressed.

We share much with our clients. We are, after all, members of the same species. What is good for them is generally good for us as well. Every so often, a client will miss a session. Seize the opportunity and hallucinate yourself into the client's chair. Imagine that you are conducting therapy with yourself. Assess your life. What would you confront yourself about? What would you recommend? Then follow your own advice. In terms of your baseline functioning, here are some of the things you would likely say.

Guard your sleep. Identify your optimal number of sleep hours, and make sure you get them, particularly on nights before seeing clients. Set a standard bedtime for yourself and keep to it in order to reduce Monday morning jet-lag sensations. Have a standard rising time as well, given that frequently staying in bed beyond your usual rising time may disrupt your circadian rhythm (Edinger & Means, 2005). Create a good sleep environment: Take note of the factors that seem to affect the quality of your sleep, and correct any that are not ideal. A coolish room temperature, heavy curtains to create cavelike darkness, a quiet environment (or a sound-smoothed one using white noise), and a comfortable bed are all invaluable. Consider sleep a foundation on which your day is built. It's worth the effort to ensure that you are rested and alert when clients walk into the clinic.

Get regular exercise. Human beings evolved to be physically active, not to sit in an ergonomically designed chair all day long. Few things seem more effective at bringing on low mood than a sedentary lifestyle. So make a point of getting at least thirty minutes of vigorous exercise at least three times each week. But do not isolate your exercise to a gym or a running track across town. Integrate physical activity into your everyday life as much as you can. Leave the car at home more often. Walk farther. Use transit, which necessitates walking to and from the stops. Eschew elevators for distances of less than three floors. Make your social life less about overeating and more about being active.

Watch your diet. Remember that most of what that nearby coffee shop sells is not really very good for you. Strive to eat a balanced diet without escaping into defeat by dwelling on the fact that you are incapable of doing so perfectly. Have breakfast. Don't wait until you are fading from hunger before you get lunch. Cut back on sugar. Use supplements when necessary.

Limit your caffeine intake. At moderate doses caffeine can sharpen a cloudy mind and banish the postlunch lull that so many people report. But it can have powerful adverse effects for a therapist. Agitation can make it difficult to sit still, stay on one topic, or tolerate a hesitant client's slow, expository manner of speaking. Impatience can tempt us to rush clients, force insights they seem slow to reach, or become frustrated with their obstinate refusal to see and agree with our viewpoints. Impulsiveness can lead us to lecture, leap off on unproductive tangents, or push directly at the client's resistance rather than slip past it. Being human, we are also prone to the other unfortunate aspects of caffeine. An hour after drinking coffee, we can find ourselves back in the muck of mental fog, craving another cup. When not seeing clients, we can find ourselves too agitated to settle into the paperwork. And if we give in to the addiction too late in the day, we can disrupt our sleep, making caffeine seem even more imperative to cut through the mist on the following day.

These are a few of what we might call foundational issues for a fulfilling life. There are others: Limit your consumption of alcohol.

Consider practicing a regular mindfulness technique, such as meditation. Convert all large and intimidating projects into a series of smaller, achievable steps. Don't work to the point of exhaustion. Create a sustainable routine in your life without imposing a suffocating rigidity.

When you find your mood slipping toward anxiety or despair, welcome the feeling. The fact that you recognize it tells you the same two things it tells your clients: you have felt this way before, and you survived it. So it can't be lethal. Use the feeling as a cue to examine your life, both the big issues (*Where am I going?*) and the routine ones (*When was the last time I exercised?*).

MAINTAIN YOUR SOCIAL NETWORK

Here's a question I often ask depressed men: "Imagine that you want to see a movie or a game, and your partner doesn't want to go. How many men do you know whom you could reasonably call up and invite to go with you?" The most frequent answer is "None." This tells us very little about men in general: most people we see in the clinic may not be thrilled with their lives. The problem is somewhat less pronounced for women, who seem to maintain and cultivate their friendships more than men do. But our culture generally tends to overvalue work and undervalue social relationships. As documented by Robert Putnam in his book *Bowling Alone: The Collapse and Revival of American Community* (2000), a decline in participation in social groups seems to be a widespread phenomenon, at least in North America.

You would think that an awareness of the value of social contact would encourage therapists to make it more of a priority in their lives, but there is little evidence to suggest this is the case. Too many clinicians seem isolated in their offices, having voluntarily adopted a role in which it is appropriate to listen to the lives of others but inappropriate to expect reciprocation. By evening, many are so emotionally exhausted that they simply collapse in front of the television or computer screen—social people becoming steadily more asocial, isolated, and dissatisfied with their lives.

Clinical work in a large organization makes social contact somewhat easier. You attend meetings, you hang out in the hallways chatting, and you have colleagues with whom you take lunch. Every so often there is a departmental social function to attend. Having had regular contact with people in multiple settings at work, it becomes easier to invite people to do things in other settings. You play squash with the guy down the hall, you go for the odd drink after work, you invite the team over for dinner, and perhaps you even date someone in the radiology department.

Private practice makes socializing more difficult. There are fewer colleagues to chat with, and you may not know the people down the hall. This makes it even more important to cultivate social contact in the rest of your life. In a previous chapter we considered strategies to enhance contact with professional colleagues. Here we must call to mind the old adage that no one reaches the end of her life wishing she had spent more time at the office. Have friends outside your work, and make spending time with them a high priority.

Let's not belabor the friend-making strategies you doubtless already suggest to lonely clients. Instead, simply remember that unless you treat your social life as an important priority in your life, it will not be satisfying, and it may wither and die. Build and defend a life in which you see friends—especially ones who have little to do with your work—several times a week. Do this, and you will have more to look back on with satisfaction in your old age than a life spent behind a desk or sitting opposite a box of tissues.

MOVE YOUR CLIENTS ONWARD

One day I finished a session with a long-term client, went back to my desk, and sat down in frustration. I had tried my best but wasn't getting anywhere. We seemed to have a good therapeutic alliance. The client developed plans to carry out between sessions and completed many of them. Nothing worked. I shifted strategies but got no further. I had seen her for thirty sessions. It occurred to me that in my entire career, I had never seen a single client who failed to improve at all in the first thirty sessions but did improve after that. I realized it was time to consider discussing the issue in depth with the client and perhaps refer her to another practitioner.

New clinicians usually assume that clients who get no benefit from therapy will stop attending. Some do, but many stay on indefinitely. I routinely get referrals of clients who have seen the same psychiatrist for ten or fifteen years: "And how much improvement have you seen in that time?" "Well, none, really." But they keep going.

Something similar can happen in your own practice. You take on ten clients. Seven get better and leave, so you take on seven more. Of that group, five get better and leave, so you take on five more, of whom four get better and leave, and so on. If you are not careful, your entire practice can become filled with nonresponders (reminiscent of the old *Bob Newhart Show*, where the psychologist kept seeing the same collection of clients season after season, none of whom ever seemed to get any better). This is discouraging for you and expensive for your clients. The truth is, you cannot help everyone who comes to see you, and you cannot rely on your clients to call a halt to an unhelpful intervention. You have to take charge.

Look at the type of therapy you offer. Is there a reasonable point at which to call it quits? If you do a short-term form of therapy for depression, at what point would you say the law of diminishing returns begins to apply? If you do an extended approach for personality disorders, doubtless your length of treatment will be longer. So if you see various populations, you might have a ballpark number of sessions in mind for each. My own policy is to set an initial contract with each client for between four and fifteen sessions and then devote a portion of a session two thirds of the way into the contract to consideration of the progress we are making. If nothing seems to be happening, we might rethink the approach, reassess to be sure the client's and my goals are in line, or consider calling a halt to the meetings. In addition, I have a fairly firm limit of thirty sessions total, which I usually tell clients about when we begin meeting. In truth,

I have sometimes seen clients for more than this number, but only when earlier results merit and only with a careful reassessment of the goals of therapy.

This said, some clients just like to have someone with whom to discuss their lives now and then. Perhaps the discussion will lead to concrete change; perhaps it will only allow the client to process his feelings. We might think of this as the haircut model of therapy: no one believes that if you get a really good haircut, you will never need another one. Psychotherapists are among the only professionals who believe that clients will come for a limited number of sessions and then maintain the benefits for the rest of their lives. If you see clients with the image of a barber in mind, then perhaps a lack of long-term change is less troubling. But even then, you should ask yourself whether you seem to be giving good haircuts. If the client is not able to take concrete steps toward change as a result of your sessions, then perhaps she is coming purely out of a misplaced hope that someday something you try will work for her. This is a path toward dependency and resentment on the part of the client, and toward burnout on the part of the therapist.

If you do not confront the issue of your nonresponders, you will go into the office each day facing a parade of your failures, your latent imposter syndrome will raise its head, and you will sit wondering when each client will see you for who you are: the Wizard of Oz, cloaked in the draperies of a therapeutic Emerald City but secretly wielding no real power.

Therapy is real, and people really do get better if we use a therapeutic approach based on sound principles and good evidence. But nothing helps everyone. Continuing to see people who do not benefit is an exercise in denial, in which our narcissistic need to believe in our own omnipotence crashes endlessly against the evidence to the contrary. It is far better to acknowledge the limitations of our powers, offer what we can, and impose reasonable limits on our work with clients. Identify nonresponders and either bring therapy to a close or refer them to a colleague who might have better luck.

ABANDON HOPE OF FRUITION

A sense of helplessness is a primary characteristic of burnout. You feel that you are banging your head against a brick wall, that you are Sisyphus, forever sentenced to push that heavy stone up the hill. One way to bring on a sense of helplessness is to be genuinely helpless: to attempt something over which you do not have control.

Therapists do this all the time. People come to see us with serious issues in their lives. They often want to hand their problems over to us, feeling that they are incapable of solving them themselves. It's tempting to take charge. We know the literature, we can see the forest despite the trees, and we do not have the client's years of momentum pushing us. As well, our self-esteem can become linked to successes with our clients. All of these factors push us in the same toxic direction: we can try to take over clients' problems, pressure them to do what we suspect will help, and hinge our own worth on the outcome.

When we try to control our clients' outcomes, this means controlling their behavior—something over which they are in charge, not us. Our resultant feeling of helplessness is neither a problem nor a distortion. We really *are* helpless. We can continue until the feeling of helplessness pervades our lives. Or we can react against the feeling by pushing these clients harder so that they submit to our will. This never works. Most client resistance is produced by excessive pressure on the part of the therapist. Clients simply refuse, "forget," or otherwise assert their independence and individuality, and fail to improve, sometimes blaming the therapist's incompetence.

What alternative is there? Should we simply give up, stop trying to help our clients, and take their money? Much depends on what we mean by "give up." If we mean that we disengage, abandon clients to their fates, and throw our hands up, then no. But if it means to refocus our efforts on what we really can control—our own behavior—then yes.

The Buddhist principle of abandoning hope of fruition is not about cultivating a sense of futility. It is about where we should direct our attention. The outcome depends to a great degree on clients' behavior. If we try to "make them behave" in a particular way, we will get pulled in an unhelpful direction. If we pull back and direct our attention to our own behavior and to the process, then we can work at being the best therapists we can be. We will be engaged with the client and will strive to deliver the best service we can. Because we are not trying to wrest control from our clients, they will have less to resist, and ultimately we will tend to have better outcomes. Further, we will accept our failures with interest and equanimity rather than self-reproach. We may become motivated to seek additional training, read more of the literature, and expand our repertoire of interventions.

RECALIBRATE YOUR TASK BALANCE

If therapy is all you do, you won't be doing it for long. For a sustainable career, you need to create a balance among various tasks. That balance is unique to you, and once you have it figured out, it will change as you go through the stages of your career. Consequently, it is worthwhile to rethink your task balance annually. You might pick your birthday, New Year's Day, September 1, or a date that bears special significance for you. Schedule it in your appointment book and keep the date. Here are some of the options to think about (a "Private-Practice Task Balancing" worksheet is available at the websites noted in the introduction):

- *Individual psychotherapy:* Don't make this a single item on your list. You probably see a variety of client populations, and you may find some (such as chronic depression) more draining than others (such as panic disorder). Split them up and contemplate your preferred numbers of each.

- *Group therapy:* Groups can be a great counterpoint to individual therapy, calling on a completely different set of skills. They typically take more preparation time and impose a greater administrative load than individual therapy, but the variety can be extremely welcome in a busy practice.

- *Assessment only:* Some clinicians hate conducting assessments—the demands for detailed reports, the interaction with third parties, the sense that the client may not be the only "customer," and in some cases the possibility of court or other procedures. Some clinicians prefer assessments over therapy: there are fewer crises, the clinician is not the primary caregiver, the emotional involvement is less intense, and it is easier to go on vacation when you don't have an ongoing treatment plan to follow. A mix of assessment-only and therapy cases can help provide balance.

- *Teaching:* A college, university, or night-school course is unlikely to make you a millionaire, but it can be a great way of helping you to organize your own thinking on a subject, and many clinicians enjoy the atmosphere of the classroom. After you have taught a class once, the preparation and revision time is usually much less, so it can become even more rewarding.

- *Clinical consultation or supervision:* Some clinicians supervise students in training or graduates applying for registration. Others provide consultation services for colleagues wanting specialty training with a particular technique or population or in private-practice development.

- *Organizational consulting:* Some clinicians provide consulting services of various sorts—for example, helping employee-assistance organizations fine-tune their services, collaborating on governmental mental health initiatives, providing guidance to businesses coping with psychological issues (such as a trauma in the workplace), or dozens of other possibilities. Consulting work of this type is usually sporadic, representing a potential way of balancing your year's activities but seldom helping to balance any given week.

- *Workshops:* Providing continuing-education programs in your specialty can be an ongoing part of a private practitioner's career. One option is to organize, promote, and host these yourself and collect your own registrations. Another is to offer the workshop to local sponsors (health regions, hospitals, nonprofits) who will do the promotion and organization for you, leaving you free to work on the actual presentation. A third is to ally with a continuing-education company, acting as one of its hired speakers.

- *Public presentations:* In addition to providing workshops for professionals, you can present talks to the general public through ongoing community talk series, community centers, or local organizations, such as churches, service clubs, or peer-support groups. These venues may or may not pay and will almost certainly not be lucrative, but they can help give you name recognition and attract clients to your clinical service.

- *Writing:* Many clinicians choose not to pursue academic careers so that they can avoid the "publish or perish" imperative. Nonacademic publishing is an attractive option for some clinicians, however. Most books do not earn enough royalties to pay well for the time spent writing them—a colleague once calculated that a paper route would be more lucrative. Publishing a book can make you a de facto expert on the topic, however, and it often pays off in name recognition and workshop presentations.

You can use any of these activities to create a task balance for your practice that will prove more sustaining than a steady diet of only one thing. In selecting them, consider the balance between diversity and synergy. The point of the exercise is to get variety into your work life, so you want the type of work you do for each activity to be different. Your career will benefit most, however, if the activities you choose work together to promote one another.

Suppose you have expertise in the treatment of anorexia nervosa. You love the clients but can't see client after client all week long, so you need something else. You could develop a continuing-education program on eating disorders that will help you organize your thoughts on the subject and give you one more reason to keep up with the literature, potentially improving the work you do with clients. You could offer public talks on the same subject, which might raise more interest in your clinical service. If you were inclined to write a book on eating disorders, you would attract many more people to your talks, and you could sell the book at the presentations. This would position you as an expert on eating disorders, making you the logical person to seek out for consultation to an in-hospital eating-disorder clinic. You will have focused your efforts on a topic of special interest to you, but you will have diversified the activities occupying your week.

However you manage your task balance, it will not remain satisfying forever. You will become more interested in writing, but your clinical load will get in the way. You will want to see more clients, but your work for the local health authority will prevent this. You will get interested in multiple projects but then feel scattered and overwhelmed. Consequently, every year take another long look at the time you spent on various activities. Ask yourself how much time you would spend on each if you could have your ideal. The ideal might prove to be too much to ask for, but notice whether there is anything within your control that will bring your annual balance into closer alignment with your aspirations. Your career is a vehicle. If you don't steer it at least once a year, who will?

PUT YOUR IDEALISM ON A LEASH

Why did you get into this field? It probably wasn't just to make money. If you are like most who wind up as therapists, you have a strong set of ideals that led you here: the desire to help (and, hidden within that admirable goal, a secret extreme: the desire to help *everyone*), the desire to change the mental health system (*completely*), the intention to reduce (no, *eliminate*) child abuse. These ideals produce enthusiasm and can drive you to study, to work hard, and to dedicate yourself to the delicate work of becoming a clinician.

Idealism is a double-edged sword, however. If you take up running to maintain your fitness, to have fun, and to participate in the odd half marathon, you'll probably keep it up for many years. If you take it up to become the world champion and keep your eye fixed on that distant goal, you will almost certainly fail, and your training sessions will be exercises in frustration. As you age, you will feel a steadily rising tide of anxiety that the dream is slipping away from you.

Let's face reality. You will not eliminate anxiety, depression, child abuse, or homelessness in your community, no matter how hard you work. You will not remake the mental health system to provide effective service to everyone who needs it. You will not create the mindful society. You will not eradicate homophobia, bigotry, sexism, or ageism. If these are your goals, you need not wait for the end of your career to discover how the story turns out. You know already. You will fail, and if you allow yourself to become fully identified with these goals, you will *be* a failure.

Idealism is a facet of narcissism. It is the belief that we are so special that we will effect massive change all on our own. Reality always defeats narcissism eventually, however. People develop an unconscious identification with a grandiose goal that is clearly beyond any single person, blinding them to contributions they have actually made: a disputed forest becomes a provincial or state park, a sponsored child in Nepal receives an education, a group of people with panic attacks experiences relief, a young woman discovers a career. To become discouraged is to suggest that these real achievements are not actually significant: the forest is irrelevant, the child does not count, the clients do not matter.

Gandhi said, "Whatever you do will be insignificant, but it is very important that you do it." Our careers will not save the planet, eradicate suffering, or create global mental health. Our names will not live on for long after our deaths. It is fine to have lofty goals. If you attach the prospect of an unrealistic and idealized outcome to your self-image, however, you will become insufferable to others, burn out, and feel like a failure.

Take some time to consider your own idealistic career goals. What would you like your work in the mental health field to accomplish? Can you think of a way of leashing this ideal, so that you can use it as your compass heading without overidentifying with the outcome? Yes, it would be nice if no one experienced anorexia to the point of requiring hospitalization. Yes, it would be terrific if no one with schizophrenia were homeless. Yes, it would be appropriate for all victims of trauma to be covered for the costs of treatment. Could you maintain that ideal while recognizing that you will not actually achieve it?

The objections to this idea are easy to anticipate: "How would any admirable goal have been achieved without idealists? We eliminated smallpox entirely and are on our way to eliminating polio. Why not believe we can create a decent mental health system or provide beds to those who need them?" Again, we can maintain our ideals while preventing them from becoming mentally toxic as we work toward them.

In my region, significant strides have been made toward environmental protection (not significant enough, in my view, but significant nevertheless). These strides were made by people working on the details of each step. Every parcel of land that has been set aside, every stream that has been preserved, every pollutant that has been curtailed—every achievement has been made by keeping the ideal of environmental preservation but working at the level of specific, achievable steps. Complete idealists may well have been involved in some of these steps, but they are unlikely to last long enough to produce genuine change.

So know your ideals. Keep them. But recognize that your contribution will most likely be to take a few steps on the journey, not to plant the flag at the summit. If you become obsessed with planting the flag, the steps you take will become unrewarding and you will eventually give up. Learn to embrace and appreciate your real achievements and your real significance, without falling prey to discouraging grandiosity.

RECLAIM YOUR UNACCEPTABLE BITS

James Hollis, in *The Middle Passage: From Misery to Meaning in Midlife* (1993), suggests that few of us are raised to be adults. We learn the ropes of childhood, and just as we are getting good at it, the rug is whipped out from under us and we are proclaimed to be adults. Naturally, we don't know how to accomplish this feat, so we look around at how other people manage it. We take the advice of parents, teachers, mentors, and the culture at large. If there is a part of us that seems unacceptable, we do our best to suppress or jettison it.

At first this strategy works well. We fit in, we get along, and we gain some real benefits: money, the esteem of others, promotions, respectability. If it seems a little unsatisfying, that's fine: we are sacrificing to build a better life somewhere off in the future. Eventually, however, we realize that we are midway through adulthood, and the fabled better life either has not materialized or has been achieved and is less than satisfying. We look in the mirror and see, with a start, that we are aging, that this *is* the future. It becomes more and more difficult to kid ourselves that we are sacrificing for a life yet to come. If we are not satisfied currently, something must change.

This is the midlife crisis, and it has two possible resolutions. We can regress toward adolescence, denying the fact that life has moved on. But this is a very temporary fix, because reality eventually returns to stamp its feet, demanding to be recognized. The other resolution is to think back, recognize the parts of ourselves that we cut away to achieve respectability and success, and reclaim them. For some this involves a complete reversal of life course, a change of career, lifestyle, relationship, home—something. For others, perhaps most, it involves a reintegration of the parts of themselves they left behind.

For example, a colleague of mine loved skiing when she was young. Eventually she went off to graduate school, and skiing vanished in the rearview mirror. Time passed, and she established herself professionally. Eventually she took up skiing again and sensed the need for renewal in her practice. She did some retraining in sports psychology and began to devote more of her work to helping competitive skiers improve their performance. Today this is a significant part of her practice, and a much-loved one.

One of the advantages of private practice is that you can, within reason, define your own work. If there is something you have always been interested in, you may be able to find a way to integrate it into your practice. You must get the appropriate training, of course, but you may already be partway there if it is an interest of yours. If you love the performing arts, you can focus your promotional efforts on that community. If you are a recreational pilot, you can ally yourself with the airlines and cultivate a subspecialty on flying phobia. If you grew up in a small town and have felt nostalgic for it ever since, you can become involved in telehealth efforts or in the provision of regional visiting clinics.

Whether you dropped a part of yourself due to a sense that it was unacceptable or because you simply couldn't see how it related to your work as a therapist, it can be worthwhile to think again. If you always wanted to run away to the circus but became a respectable clinician instead, you don't have to abandon your career and learn the trapeze at age forty. But you can still become a preferred provider for an entertainment company like Cirque du Soleil. One of the keys to avoiding burnout is to identify your true passions, especially the ones you have left unexplored, and find a way to bring them back into your life—either professionally or through an avocation.

ASK THE CRISP QUESTION ANNUALLY

Quentin Crisp was a flamboyantly gay Englishman who spent most of his working life as an artist's model for government postsecondary institutions, a profession that inspired the title of his biography: *The Naked Civil Servant* (1968). At age seventy-two he moved to New York City, lived in a small room in lower Manhattan, reviewed movies, wrote many more books, inspired Sting's song "Englishman in New York," played Queen Elizabeth in the movie *Orlando*, and performed in his one-man show *An Evening with Quentin Crisp*.

Crisp's philosophy is perhaps best indicated by his suggestion of the most important question in life: "Ask yourself, 'If there were no praise, and no blame, who would I be then?' Then you know who you are, and what your style is" (as quoted in Fountain, 2002, p. 115). In other words, how would you live your life if you eliminated activities designed to elicit the admiration or avoid the disapproval of others?

It's tempting to discard the question as sociopathic. If others didn't count, perhaps we would live selfish, hedonistic lives, wreaking havoc all around us and ending up miserable. Crisp himself, however, was unfailingly polite; he was a clear and independent thinker who died at ninety, beloved by most who knew him. His point was that living your life in order to be acceptable in the eyes of others leads not to happiness but to conformity, blandness, and frustration borne of psychic self-suffocation. Given the titanic forces of conformity arrayed around each of us, the erection of a firm bulwark of self-determination is almost essential.

One of the causes of burnout for many professionals can be this relentless eroding of the self in the service of your role. Even the idea of "looking professional" can entail submerging your individuality to project a certain societally approved image. Psychotherapists, in particular, deliberately set aside their own issues and concerns to be fully present for the client's presence and personality—some of us striving to become Freud's blank screen, others attempting merely to respond accurately to what the client brings in, without distorting too much based on our own history or cognitive peccadilloes.

I have earlier advocated an annual task rebalancing: an assessment of the current distribution of our energies across the various professional tasks and roles available to us. Here let us add to this a panoramic scope that takes in not only our careers but also our lives in total. Use the brainstorming strategy of setting aside the constraints of reality and social convention, and ask yourself the Crisp question about your life. If you couldn't impress anyone, and if no one really cared what you did, what would you do? Or, if this works better for you, ask, "What would I be doing if I took my life seriously?" or "… if my life actually mattered?"

The Long View: Burnout and Beyond

Asking the question is not the same as signing a contract. Perhaps your answers will scare you. You might leave your marriage, close your clinic, live in a hut in Bali, tell certain members of your family just what you think of them, or spend your retirement savings. And someday, perhaps you really will do some or all of these things. Having asked the question, keep it open until you come up with at least a few things you are willing to consider. Several times over the next few decades, you will probably start a revolution in your life, or you will have one thrust on you. Perhaps opening a private practice (and reading this book) is part of one such shift. Regardless, at least once a year, sit back, take the broad view, look where your sailboat is headed, ask yourself whether that is really where you want to be going, and act on at least part of the answer.

CULTIVATE AN AVOCATION

Is it any wonder that people have such difficulty establishing and maintaining relationships when we spend our youth listening to music that endlessly repeats myths about love? One of the most pernicious ideas is *You'll be my everything*: if you find the right partner, that person will satisfy your every need and share your every interest. Believing such a notion will lead inevitably to disappointment. No one will be our everything, ever. We will always need other people in our lives, and recognizing this fact will help to maintain our relationships.

Work is similar. Job finders and ill-trained life coaches inform you that there is a job out there with your name on it, and that when you find it, you will be endlessly excited to go to work. You will bound out of bed every morning, thrilled at the privilege of having your job. You will be joyful at every task, admired universally for your skills.

But you won't. No job will counter the effects of incipient flu, a bad night's sleep, or the fight you had yesterday with your spouse. No job provides relentless excitement or meshes perfectly with our needs and personalities. There is always some part of us that is unfulfilled; there are always some tasks we find tedious or certain days we would rather play hooky. If we are reasonably well suited to our work, we will be interested more often than not, we will feel lucky when we compare ourselves to at least some of our friends, and we will genuinely look forward to at least some of the tasks before us. The expectation of continuous rapt engagement, however, is bound to produce discontent.

To be sustainably fulfilled, we must have something else in our lives: friends, exercise, leisure—and, for many of us, an avocation, something vaguely worklike that fulfills a part of us that our regular jobs cannot reach.

There is another reason to cultivate an avocation. Clinical practice can be fulfilling, but it has some disadvantages. You never really accomplish anything. You don't actually cure people. The best you can do is lay the groundwork for clients to cure themselves. When they do get better, you can never really tell whether it was your own efforts that counted. Perhaps they would have gotten better with the simple passage of time. If you do assessment-only work, all you really do is attempt to understand the problem and perhaps put a label on it. You don't change anything at all.

This disconnect between effort and result is not unique to clinical work. Lawyers push paper and talk, but produce nothing. Physicians make suggestions that patients may or may not follow, and every patient dies eventually no matter what they do. Architects draw pictures and rely on others to create buildings. Engineers design things, but laborers do most of the work. Broadcasters talk. Journalists type. Most urban workers don't produce anything tangible and often wonder if they make any impact at all: *If I weren't here to do this work, would anyone really notice?* Learned helplessness theory (Abramson, Seligman, & Teasdale, 1978) suggests that depression is a natural consequence of an environment in which the link between your own behavior and tangible outcomes breaks down. Much modern work has precisely this quality.

For these reasons, most of us need to have other interests that complement our work lives. Your avocational interest should be something quite different from your regular employment. Doing therapy

The Long View: Burnout and Beyond

all day and providing pro bono therapy for a charity two evenings a week will not usually do. If your vocation and avocation are too similar, you will either give up the avocation or be more, not less, likely to burn out. The avocation should represent an interest your regular work cannot fulfill.

An avocation may or may not produce revenue. The word itself makes clear that this is *not* your vocation, not your source of funds. Considering activities that do not produce revenue can significantly widen your horizon. Perhaps no one is ever going to pay to see you and your buddies perform with your garage band. Fine. Your professional work will pay the bills.

Given the ephemerality of therapy practice, most therapists would be well advised to choose an avocation that produces tangible results. Volunteering for an advisory board may be fine for some, but it may resemble too closely the indirect, advisory role of a therapist. When I surveyed clinicians about their avocations, several themes emerged:

- *Creativity:* Although clinical work is a collaboration between two people, it is essentially all about the client. (That's why the client pays us, rather than the other way around.) Many clinicians have avocations that emphasize personal expression through music, writing, or visual arts. Some people play in musical groups or sing in choirs. One therapist I asked has a sideline in wedding photography, another in Web design. Several write fiction.

- *Action:* Therapy is sedentary and quiet. A complementary activity can be something more action oriented. One colleague is a wilderness guide; another leads travel groups through Asia. A former mentor of mine races stock cars and gives training to other enthusiasts in competitive driving. A good friend has trained as a mahout (an elephant handler) and supports an elephant refuge in Thailand.

- *Product:* A colleague who doubles as a carpenter points out that when he builds a cabinet, there is no debate about who created it or whether the wood might have formed itself into a cabinet without him. There is a visible product that can be used, touched, and experienced.

When my partner and I decided to look for a cottage outside town, we did not have an avocation in mind. We looked at various properties, but none seemed quite right, so we finally gave up. Four days after making that decision, a friend called to say he saw a place for sale near his own property. We stayed at his house for the weekend and, early one morning, went to take a look at what turned out to be an operating orchard and farm. Neither of us had ever expressed an interest in farming, but otherwise the place had everything we were looking for: isolation, ample room for guests, office space, water access, a local community—everything. We looked at each other and decided within half an hour to buy it.

We got an avocation in the process, one that turned out to suit us well. Today we produce six types of fruit, host friends for weekends, offer the place for writers' retreats, and spend our time on physical tasks that bear tangible results: fruit grown, fences mended, lawns mowed, equipment repaired. Much of this book was written there, between farm chores.

An avocation gives you an extra support in your life. If your practice is not going so well, perhaps your apple crop is abundant. If the art show doesn't produce sales, perhaps your referral rate is up. If a client is frustrating you, you can go home and work in the wood shop. No job will be your everything. So have an affair behind its back. Get an avocation, and make it as different from your work life as you can.

LISTEN TO THE WHISPERS OF BURNOUT

Perhaps in reading this chapter, you are hoping burnout will never happen to you. This is the wrong approach. It will almost certainly happen; the only question is to what degree and what you will do about it.

Many clients use a binary question when it comes to coping: *Can I still handle it—yes or no?* If yes, then they stay the course and keep going. If no, then they come to therapy or stop coping entirely. Some clients worry that their problems indicate that they have weak personalities. In fact, it is often the stronger ones who wind up in real trouble. If they were weaker, they would have been forced to change course much earlier, before the problem became truly intractable.

So stop hoping you will never burn out. Recognize that burnout is a continuum, not a dichotomy, and that, as with every continuum, you are already on it. The trick is not to close your eyes and pray you will never reach the far pole. Instead, watch carefully for the early signs of burnout and intervene before they worsen.

Perhaps you already know what happens to you when you are nearing the edge. Perhaps you drink more coffee or become cynical. Perhaps you push your clients too hard and start getting more resistance. Perhaps you begin to sense that you are working harder than they are. Perhaps your billing falls behind, or you get irritable with your partner. Perhaps you start working longer hours. Perhaps you start leaving your session notes for longer and longer periods before completing them. Perhaps you go for weeks without calling your friends. Perhaps burnout happens when you neglect your fitness, or when it's been too long since your last vacation. Perhaps you start feeling exhausted in the evenings, unable to do anything other than flip on the television. Perhaps you feel under constant time pressure, plotting how you can possibly get everything done in the day. Perhaps you begin to reflect that your depressed clients may be right to view life as negatively as they do. Perhaps a general sense of gray flatness begins to pervade your life, extinguishing joy and laughter, dulling your libido, and making none of the activities that would normally give you pleasure seem appealing.

Take a moment to think about the last time you came close to burnout. What happened? What were the external circumstances? How did you feel? How did your behavior change? (A "Your Burnout Warning Signs" worksheet on this issue is available at the websites noted in the introduction.)

Stop thinking of these circumstances, feelings, and behaviors as enemies or threats, and start valuing them for what they are: your guides. These are the signposts that say you are on the road to burnout. If you could welcome them, if you could listen to what they have to tell you, perhaps you could catch yourself and change course earlier the next time they appear. Once again, this involves using knowledge we routinely give our clients: pay attention, look at the signposts, know where they lead, and place your hand on the tiller. You need never find yourself in the midst of burnout. There are always warnings. All we have to do is pay attention to them.

PLAN YOUR RETIREMENT

Private practice affords a golden opportunity to plan your retirement sanely, unlike a career spent working for a major institution. You can, if you wish, work full-time right up until an arbitrary birthday, then slam on the brakes, pack up your desk, and attempt to shift the momentum of the past thirty years in a single day.

If you do this, your fantasy of retirement will risk being guided by the activities that have been crowded out by your work demands. You never had time to travel, so now you imagine you will drive the roads endlessly in an RV. You never had time to golf, so in retirement you think the "golfing lifestyle" advertised on curbside real estate signs sounds lovely. Then you will play golf daily for a week or two before getting bored and realizing you have made a profound mistake, trading your overdose of work for an overdose of your fantasy rather than striving for a new balance. The RV will become a prison and the open road a rootless nightmare, a Sisyphean chore to drive.

Most private practitioners shift their work in increments over time. They may drop to four days a week, then three days plus teaching a college course; then they may close their practices in summer to travel. They may gradually reduce the number of people they see each day, renting out their spaces to others for a bit more and a bit more. As the gaps that used to be occupied by clinical work grow, they are gradually filled with what has been lacking. You wanted to golf more; now you can golf on Wednesday afternoons. This satisfies your golfing hunger, so that you avoid the trap of buying a home beside the golf course and can devote the next gap to another long-held desire. You take three weeks off every few months, which allows you to go off in your RV to your heart's content—no need to overbalance by selling the home base.

This way of making the transition mimics the gradual approach people have taken for centuries. The hunter gradually morphs into a leader, then into an elder who might occasionally take the grandchildren out onto the land, but without the pressure of providing a full measure of the community's diet. The way we have come to think of retirement—as a single, wrenching life change—is unhelpful and, to a great extent, unnatural. Over thirty or forty years of working, you build up tremendous inertial momentum; it is unrealistic to expect to turn your life on a dime on your sixty-fifth birthday.

Many of us never want to retire if, by retirement, we mean abandoning the field entirely, along with all of our hard-won expertise. The rocking chair may occasionally seem attractive, but we are all too aware that it would quickly become dull, leaving us with a feeling of meaninglessness. Our work lives will certainly change, but by degrees, so that perhaps we will work well into our eighties, but not in a clinic or strapped into a consulting-room chair. We may shift our emphasis to writing, to committee work for the local professional organization, or to advocacy. We may even go on seeing clients, perhaps a day a week, perhaps a half day. As the fields of our lives are gradually taken out of clinical production, we will plant other crops, some related to our professional lives, some not. We will retire naturally and with forethought—if we plan wisely.

Postscript

In his excellent book *The Pleasures and Sorrows of Work* (2009), Alain de Botton reflects on the fragmentation of production in modern workplaces. Whereas once a person might collect ingredients, bake, and serve a tea biscuit, in a modern food corporation the tasks involved have been sliced so thinly that it becomes difficult for workers to take personal pride in the product or to feel that they are engaged in meaningful and elevating work. Although twenty-first-century methods of organizing work have led to tremendous wealth and to gains in the material standard of living, they may have imposed the cost of alienation.

Opening a private psychotherapy practice reverses the centuries-long trend toward specialization and creates a more human-scaled cottage industry, one with the inevitable inefficiencies of small business, but one that has the potential for much greater satisfaction for those employed in it. Outcomes are clearly tied to efforts. Clients are seen by the same person from assessment through to follow-up. Decisions about populations to see, hours of operation, modalities used, and all other aspects of clinic operation are adopted intentionally, not imposed by others. Although anxiety producing, due to the necessity of performing tasks for which we are not trained, private practice does not typically create the feeling of being a cog in a large and impersonal machine.

Clinical work is difficult. Life is inherently complicated, and pain is an inevitable component of it. We will all have our problems, clinicians and clients alike. We will not cure, or even help, everyone who comes to see us, and much of what we say may seem to have little or no impact.

In 1989, the *Exxon Valdez* ran aground in Prince William Sound, Alaska, spilling millions of gallons of crude oil from its cargo tanks. The vessel was so large that turning the wheel would initially seem to produce no effect; it took several kilometers to execute a turn. Clients appear, at first glance, to be much more maneuverable. Surely our work should have a more-or-less immediate effect. Not so.

Stay in the field long enough, and eventually a client will return or greet you on the street. The person will thank you for the time you spent with her and for the changes she brought about in her life as a result. She will say, "The most important thing was your story about the apple." You will smile vaguely. And you will think, *I don't remember any story about an apple.* She will say, "It has stayed with me all this time and has made such a difference in my life." And you will realize that sometime, four years ago, you helped this person turn the wheel. Perhaps you thought of this client as one of your failed efforts. But it just took a little longer for the enormity of her life to begin to change course.

Counseling, coaching, and psychotherapy are good fields. Taken seriously and practiced with integrity, they are honorable professions. Some of our greatest successes we will never know about. When I bought the orchard, I found a crochet hook in the barn. Not being one to crochet, I nearly tossed it out. Then I learned that it was the perfect shape to clear sprinkler heads of the debris that clogs them. What at first seemed so small and insignificant turned out to be one of the most valuable tools on the farm.

In every field there are tricks, shortcuts, and useful tools. Many of them are not obvious from the outset. With time, we learn some and invent others. In this book I have tried to present some of the ideas that have helped me. Perhaps you will find a crochet hook among them. I hope so. Good luck.

Running a private practice is endlessly detailed, and no single book can encompass all of the issues. This book has attempted to cover a broad range of ideas on the topic, but doubtless, hundreds have been missed. If you have ideas for subsequent editions of this book, please write me at paterson@changeways.com. I would be glad to hear from you.

References

Abramson, L. Y., Seligman, M. E., & Teasdale, J. D. (1978). Learned helplessness in humans: Critique and reformulation. *Journal of Abnormal Psychology, 87*(1), 49–74.

American Psychological Association (APA) Committee on Legal Issues. (2006). Strategies for private practitioners coping with subpoenas or compelled testimony for client records or test data. *Professional Psychology: Research and Practice, 37*(2), 215–222.

Chilton, D. (1989). *The wealthy barber: The common sense guide to successful financial planning.* Toronto: Stoddart Publishing Company.

Crisp, Q. (1968). *The naked civil servant.* New York: HarperCollins.

Crisp, Q., & Carroll, D. (1981). *Doing it with style.* London: Methuen.

De Botton, A. (2009). *The pleasures and sorrows of work.* New York: Pantheon Books.

Dewa, C. S., Chau, N., & Dermer, S. (2010). Examining the comparative incidence and costs of physical and mental health-related disabilities in an employed population. *Journal of Occupational and Environmental Medicine, 52*(7), 758–762.

Edinger, J. D., & Means, M. K. (2005). Cognitive-behavioral therapy for primary insomnia. *Clinical Psychology Review, 25*(5), 539–558.

Fountain, T. (2002). *Quentin Crisp.* Bath, UK: Absolute Press.

Fredrickson, B. L. (2009). *Positivity: Groundbreaking research reveals how to embrace the hidden strength of positive emotions, overcome negativity, and thrive.* New York: Crown Publishers.

Fredrickson, B. L., & Losada, M. F. (2005). Positive affect and the complex dynamics of human flourishing. *American Psychologist, 60*(7), 678–686.

Heider, F. (1958). *The psychology of interpersonal relations.* New York: John Wiley & Sons.

Hollis, J. (1993). *The middle passage: From misery to meaning in midlife.* Toronto: Inner City Books.

Koch, W. J. (2009). Personal communication.

Koocher, G. P., & Keith-Spiegel, P. (2008). *Ethics in psychology and the mental health professions: Standards and cases.* New York: Oxford University Press.

Paterson, R. J. (2000). *The assertiveness workbook: How to express your ideas and stand up for yourself at work and in relationships.* Oakland, CA: New Harbinger Publications.

Putnam, R. D. (2000). *Bowling alone: The collapse and revival of American community.* New York: Simon & Schuster.

Tracy, B. (2001). *Eat that frog! 21 great ways to stop procrastinating and get more done in less time.* San Francisco, CA: Berrett-Koehler Publishers.

Turcotte, M. (2006). General social survey on time use: Cycle 19—The time it takes to get to work and back 2005. Statistics Canada, catalogue no. 89-622-XIE.

U.S. Census Bureau. (2005). Americans spend more than 100 hours commuting to work each year, Census Bureau reports. American Community Survey (ACS), March 30. http://www.census.gov/newsroom/releases/archives/american_community_survey_acs/cb05-ac02.html

Randy J. Paterson, PhD, owns and operates Changeways Clinic, a private multiple-provider outpatient practice in Vancouver, British Columbia. He is author of *The Assertiveness Workbook* and *Your Depression Map*. Through Changeways Clinic, he presents lectures and workshops internationally on topics including mental health policy, cognitive behavioral therapy, the nature and treatment of depression and anxiety disorders, and strategies for private practice management. He was the 2008 recipient of the Canadian Psychological Association's Distinguished Practitioner Award. For more information on Paterson, his presentations and workshops, or Changeways Clinic, visit www.changeways.com.

Index

A

abbreviation system, 130, 131–132
accessibility of services, 9; office location and, 39; wheelchair accessibility, 45
accountants, 154–155
active avocations, 243
active vs. inactive files, 133
addresses, website, 97–98
administrative demands, 20
adolescent clients, 30–31
adult clients, 30
advance package, 186–188
age groups, 30–31
age of consent, 119
agency referral lists, 86–88
American Psychological Association, 125
animated websites, 106
announcement letter, 82–83

anxiety: about asking for fees, 22–23; about terminating assistants, 167
artwork on websites, 106
Assertiveness Workbook, The (Paterson), 175
assessments: assessment-only practice, 37, 233; factors involved in, 189–190; setting standard times for, 181–182; time requirements for, 182–184
assistants, 161–177; assigning tasks to, 168–169, 173–174; calculating hours needed from, 162–163; clinic manual written by, 165; costs of replacing, 170; employer role related to, 171–173; feedback ratio for, 174–175; hiring friends as, 165–168; needlessly apologizing to, 173–174; offering raises to, 170–171; providing

corrective feedback to, 175–177; systematizing tasks for, 163–164
automobile insurers, 87
avocational interests, 242–244

B

balance theory, 83–84
base salary, 144–149
bathrooms, office, 45, 48, 63
behavioral goals, 190
benefits packages, 24, 158–159
big-organization hassles, 6–8
blogs, 108–109
book publishing, 234
booking appointments, 194–196
bookshelves, 57, 62
Bowling Alone: The Collapse and Revival of American Community (Putnam), 227
brainstorming, 216–217
brochures/pamphlets, 66, 77–79
browser test, 108
buildings: qualities of office, 44–46; wheelchair accessibility of, 45
burnout prevention, 225–247; avocational interests and, 242–244; basic guidelines for, 225–227; Crisp question and, 239–241; directing attention for, 231–232; idealism and, 235–237; reclaiming parts of yourself for, 238–239; recognizing signs of burnout for, 244–246; retirement transition and, 246–247; social contact and, 227–228; task balance and, 232–235; therapeutic relationship and, 228–230. *See also* sustainability considerations
business cards, 65–66
business issues: clerical demands, 19–20; defining your business product, 75–76; home vs. business accounts, 144; registering for applicable taxes, 157–158; structuring your business, 155–157. *See also* financial issues
business licenses, 158

C

caffeine intake, 226
calculators, 67
Capreol, Martha, 218
career goals, 237
carpeting floors, 55
ceiling of office, 48, 54, 56
chairs, office, 57, 193
changeways.com website, 2
children, working with, 31
Chilton, David, 160
cleaning: of client files, 134; of office space, 49
clerical issues/demands, 19–20
clients: access to services, 9; active vs. inactive, 133; advance package for, 186–188; age groups of, 30–31; chairs used by, 57; cleaning out files for, 134; color coding files for, 128; computer security related to, 134–136; consent to treatment form, 120–121; demographic information form, 115–118; exclusionary factors, 34–35; fear of not getting, 17; freedom to choose, 10; limits to confidentiality form, 119–120; load capacity for seeing, 185–186; managing information about, 113–136; number assignments, 114–115; organizing files of, 129; release of information form, 118; requests for information about, 125–127; session notes about, 122–125, 129–132; specific populations of,

31–33; therapeutic relationship with, 228–230; vacation tips related to, 214–215
clinic assistants. *See* assistants
clinic manual, 165
clinical services, 179–198; advance package, 186–188; assessment times and, 181–184; client load considerations, 185–186; dealing with bookings and payment, 194–196; initial intake process, 188–190; in-office vacations and, 184–185; planning your week for, 180–181; preparing the office space for, 192–194; session planning process, 191–192; setting therapy goals, 190–191; ten-minute rule, 196–197; writing session notes, 197–198
clinical trial research groups, 86
clocks in office, 61
closed-ended groups, 35
clothing tips, 68–73; for men, 72–73; for women, 71–72
coaches, 211
coatrack in office, 63–64
collegial relationships, 20–21, 209–211
color coding files, 128
commuting to work, 15
competence issues, 119
computer security issues, 134–136
conferences, 211–212
confidentiality: computer security and, 134–136; limits to confidentiality form, 119–120
consent to treatment form, 120–121
consultation: clinician groups for, 210; providing to organizations, 233; supervision and, 210, 233
consumer advocacy organizations, 110

contact info on website, 112
continuing-education events, 211–212, 234
corrective feedback, 175–177
corresponding with referral sources, 91–92
couples therapy, 120
creative avocations, 243
Crisp, Quentin, 70, 239–240
customer-centered perspective, 10

D

daybooks, 204
de Botton, Alain, 249
de Chamfort, Nicolas, 202
degrees/qualifications, 60
demographic information form, 115–118
depression, 242
designing your website: elements to avoid in, 106; hiring a designer for, 106–107; preparations required for, 102–105. *See also* website creation
desk in office, 57, 193, 215
dietary habits, 226
directory listings, 85–86
disability insurers, 87
distress, medical model of, 8–9
Doing It with Style (Crisp), 70
doors of office/suite, 47, 54–55

E

electronic letterhead, 66
e-mail checking, 203
employees: employer role related to, 171–173; hiring friends as, 165–168; offering raises to, 170–171; providing feedback to, 174–177. *See also* assistants
employer role, 171–173
encrypted flash drives, 135–136

Ethics in Psychology and the Mental Health Professions (Koocher and Keith-Spiegel), 125
exclusionary factors, 34–35
exercise, 225–226
expenses: limiting ongoing, 153–154; paid from income, 139–140; tax deductible, 142–143
exposure therapy, 22
exterior signage, 64
Exxon Valdez analogy, 250

F

family therapy, 120
fantasies of private practice, 6–16
fax machines, 67
fears of private practice, 16–27
feedback: effective wording of corrective, 175–177; ratio of positive vs. negative, 174–175
file cabinets, 57–58
files: active vs. inactive, 133; cleaning out, 134; color coding, 128; computer security for, 134–136; organizing, 129
financial issues, 137–160; benefits package, 24, 158–159; business structure, 155–156; charging for actual time, 140–142; determining therapy fees, 138–140; hiring an accountant, 154–155; holiday/vacation costs, 13, 212; home vs. business accounts, 144; incorporation, 156–157; lifestyle choices, 150–151; overhead expenses, 139–140, 153–154; paying yourself a base salary, 144–149; realistic approach to, 151–152; retirement plan, 24, 159–160; salaried vs. private practice, 11–12, 138–140; sliding fee scale, 152–153; taxes, 142–143, 157–158. *See also* income considerations
first session note, 122–124
flash drives, 135–136
flexible work hours, 13–15
flip charts, 58–60
floor coverings, 55
forms: consent to treatment, 120–121; demographic information, 115–118; limits to confidentiality, 119–120; referral, 79–81; release of information, 118; website for downloadable, 2
formulation, 123–124
Fredrickson, Barbara, 175
friends: importance of contact with, 228; problems with hiring, 165–168
furniture: office, 56–58; waiting room, 63

G

Gandhi, Mohandas K., 236
Gilliam, Terry, 7
goal setting, 190–191
group therapy, 34–35, 232

H

health insurance, 159
health maintenance organizations (HMOs), 87
heating/cooling systems, 47
helplessness, feelings of, 231
hiring people: accountant, 154–155; clinic assistant, 161–177; website designer, 106–107
holidays. *See* vacations/holidays
Hollis, James, 238
home offices, 40–42; advantages/disadvantages of, 40–41; home-to-work transition in, 201; zoning laws related to, 41–42

home page of website, 101–102
home-to-work transition, 200–201
human resources departments, 87–88
humor, importance of, 3

I

idealism, 235–237
inactive files, 133
income considerations: charging for actual time, 140–142; determining therapy fees, 138–140; expenses paid from income, 139–140, 153–154; lifestyle choices and, 150–151; paying yourself a base salary, 144–149; realistic approach to, 151–152; requesting payment from clients, 22–23, 194–196; salaried vs. private practice, 11–12, 138–140; sliding fee scale and, 152–153; supplementing salaried income, 12–13; tax deductible expenses and, 142–143; uncertainty about monthly income, 18–19. *See also* financial issues
income tax, 157
incorporation, 156–157
individual psychotherapy, 34, 232
information about clients: demographic information, 115–118; handling requests for, 125–127
information forms: consent to treatment, 120–121; demographic information, 115–118; limits to confidentiality, 119–120; release of information, 118
in-office vacations, 184–185
insurers: charging for reports to, 141–142; private practice referrals from, 23–24; requests for information from, 125–127
intake process, 188–190
interior signage, 64–65
Internet resources. *See* Web-based resources

J

joint partnership, 155–156

K

Keith-Spiegel, Patricia, 125
keywords, website, 111
Koch, William, 126
Koocher, Gerald, 125

L

lamps for office, 58
lawyers: charging for reports to, 141–142; requests for information from, 125–127
learned helplessness theory, 242
lease agreement, 50–51
legal issues: confidentiality and, 119–120; requests for information, 125–127
leisure at work, 205–206
letterhead, 66
liability issues, 156–157
lifestyle resources, 110
lighting, office, 193
limits to confidentiality form, 119–120
links page on website, 109–110
list making, 204–205
location of office, 39–40
logo/design for business, 65
long-term therapy, 38
lunch dates, 207, 210

M

magazines in waiting room, 64

mail checking rituals, 203
maintenance of office space:
    questions to ask about, 49; rental rate plus fee for, 50, 51
management: of business finances, 137–160; of client information, 113–136; of clinical services, 179–198
marketing and promotion: agency referral lists for, 86–88; directory listings for, 85–86; pamphlets/brochures for, 77–79; private-practice announcement for, 82–83; product definition for, 75–76; referral networks for, 88–89; reluctance to embrace, 17–18
medical model of distress, 8–9
men, clothing tips for, 72–73
mental health information sites, 109, 110
mentors, 211
Middle Passage: From Misery to Meaning in Midlife, The (Hollis), 238
midlife crisis, 238
money issues. *See* financial issues
music in waiting room, 63

N

Naked Civil Servant, The (Crisp), 239
naming your practice, 35–37
narcissism, 236
navigating websites, 107–108
neighborhood considerations, 39–40
networking: events devoted to, 89; referral network created for, 88; reluctance to practice, 17–18
nonclinical administrators, 7
note taking: after sessions, 197–198; first session notes, 122–124; ongoing session notes, 124–125; personal system for, 129–132
number assignments, 114–115

O

office space, 39–51; asking tenants about, 49–50; building considerations, 44–46; carpeting floor of, 55; ceiling of, 48, 54, 56; client's view of, 61–62; clocks placed in, 61; degrees/qualifications displayed in, 60; electronic components in, 66–67; furniture in, 56–58; home-based, 40–42; lease agreement for, 50–51; neighborhood considerations, 39–40; olfactory environment, 73–74; preparing before sessions, 192–194; serviced or turnkey, 42–44; signage related to, 64–65; soundproofing, 54–55; stationery used in, 65–66; suite considerations, 46–49; waiting room, 46–47, 62–65; walls and windows of, 48, 55–56; whiteboard or flip chart in, 58–60
olfactory environment, 73–74
ongoing session notes, 124–125
open-ended groups, 35
optimism, 151–152
organizational consulting, 233
organizational issues: big-organization hassles, 6–7; client accessibility limitations, 9; medical model of distress, 8
organizing client files, 129
overhead expenses, 153–154

P

pamphlets, 77–79

pay rates: private practice income and, 144–149; salaried vs. private practice, 11; sliding fee scale and, 152–153. *See also* income considerations
payroll taxes, 157–158
performance-based raises, 171
phone system, 66
physical exercise, 225–226
planning: clinical schedule, 180–181; retirement, 24, 159–160, 246–247
playing at work, 205–206
Pleasures and Sorrows of Work, The (de Botton), 249
point-of-sale terminal, 67
positive thinking, 151
Positivity (Fredrickson), 175
practice updates, 92
preferred provider organizations (PPOs), 87
presentation costs, 140–141
printers/fax machines, 67
prioritizing referral sources, 92–93
private practice: announcement letter, 82–83; arguments in favor of, 6–16; assessment and therapy in, 37–38; assistants used in, 161–177; balancing your work load in, 25–26; basing on personal vision, 15–16; benefit packages in, 24, 158–159; burnout prevention in, 225–247; clerical and business demands of, 19–20; client accessibility and choice in, 9–10; clothing tips for clinicians in, 68–73; collegial relationships in, 20–21, 209–211; defining your business for, 75–76; exclusionary factors in, 33–34; expenses and reimbursements in, 138–140; fears and arguments against, 16–27; group vs. individual therapy in, 34–35; income considerations related to, 11–12, 18–19, 137–160; information management in, 113–136; maintaining a sense of meaning in, 26–27; managing clinical services in, 179–198; marketing and promotion of, 17–18; naming guidelines for, 35–37; office space for, 39–51, 53–67, 73–74; referrals in, 23–24, 76–93; requesting payment in, 22–23, 194–196; retirement planning in, 24, 159–160, 246–247; rituals and sustainability in, 199–221; short-term vs. long-term therapy in, 38; supplementing salaried income with, 12–13; transitioning to retirement from, 246–247; vacations/holidays from, 13–14, 212–217; website creation for, 95–112; work schedule flexibility in, 13–15
private-practice announcement, 82–83
productive avocations, 243–244
productivity initiatives, 7
professional organizations: benefits packages offered by, 159; providing website links to, 110; referral services offered by, 85
promotion. *See* marketing and promotion
public presentations, 234
publicly funded clinics, 86
publishing books, 234
Putnam, Robert, 227

Q

qualifications/degrees, 60

R

raises: giving to yourself, 149; offering to assistants, 170–171
recording appointments, 204
referrals, 75–93; agency lists and, 86–88; colleague lists and, 88; corresponding with sources of, 91–92; defining your product for, 75–76; directory listings and, 85–86; fear of not getting, 17; form for obtaining, 79–81; freedom to decline, 23–24; identifying sources of, 76–77; keeping a book of, 89–90; networking events and, 89; pamphlet for cultivating, 77–79; prioritizing your sources of, 92–93; private-practice announcements and, 82–83; referring to sources of, 83–84; returning calls about, 90–91; thank-you notes for, 91; Web-based services for, 85
regulations, 7
reimbursements, 138–139
release of information form, 118
rental rate for office, 50, 51
requests for information, 125–127
retirement plans, 24, 159–160, 246–247
rituals, 199–221; collegial contact, 209–211; continuing-education, 211–212; getting out of the office, 206–207; home-to-work transition, 200–201; importance of structure and, 199–200; life-work balance, 217–219; play/leisure at work, 205–206; responding to project requests, 219–220; scheduling and list-making, 204–205; unpleasant task fulfillment, 202; vacation strategies and, 212–217; voice-mail and e-mail checking, 203; work-to-home transition, 207–209
role resistance, 166
routine tasks, 163–164

S

sailing metaphors, 223–224
salaried income: paying yourself a base salary, 144–149; private practice income compared to, 11–12; supplementing through private practice, 12–13
sales taxes, 158
savings plan, 159–160
scents in office, 73–74
scheduling issues: planning your clinical week, 180–181; private practice flexibility and, 13–15; recording appointments, 204
search engine results, 111
seasonal cards, 91–92
security: of computer files, 134–136; of office space, 47
self-promotion, 18
seniors, working with, 30
serviced office space, 42–44; advantages/disadvantages of, 42–43; recommendations on choosing, 44
session notes: first session, 122–124; ongoing sessions, 124–125; system for taking, 129–132; writing after sessions, 197–198
short-term therapy, 38
sick days, 159
side tables in office, 58
signage, exterior/interior, 64–65
sink in office suite, 48–49
size of office space, 46–47
sleep habits, 225
sliding fee scale, 152–153

social contact, 227–228
social service information, 110
sole proprietorship, 155
soundproofing, 54–55
special populations, 31–33
stationery, 65–66
storage unit, 58
suffixes, website, 98
suites, office, 46–49
superego poisoning, 217
supervision: consultation and, 210, 233; employer role of, 171–173; friends and resistance to, 167
sustainability considerations, 199–221; collegial contact, 209–211; continuing-education events, 211–212; getting out of the office, 206–207; home-to-work transition, 200–201; life-work balance, 217–219; personal rituals and, 199–200; play/leisure at work, 205–206; responding to project requests, 219–220; scheduling and list-making, 204–205; unpleasant task fulfillment, 202; vacation strategies, 212–217; voice-mail and e-mail checking, 203; work-to-home transition, 207–209. *See also* burnout prevention

T

tasks: accomplishing unpleasant, 202; assigning to assistants, 168–169; creating a balance among, 232–235; systematizing routine, 163–164
taxes: deducting expenses from, 142–143; hiring an accountant for, 154–155; incorporated businesses and, 156; registering for applicable, 157–158

teaching classes, 233
temperature of office, 193
ten-minute rule, 196–197
termination anxiety, 167
thank-you notes, 91
therapeutic relationship, 228–230
therapy: advance package for, 186–188; assessment offered with, 37–38, 233; clinician use of, 210; consent to treatment form, 120–121; fees charged for, 138–140; group vs. individual, 34–35; intake assessment for, 188–190; limits to confidentiality in, 119–120; preparing the office space for, 192–194; session planning for, 191–192; setting goals for, 190–191; short-term vs. long-term, 38; ten-minute rule in, 196–197. *See also* clinical services
Tracy, Brian, 202
turnkey offices, 42–44; advantages/disadvantages of, 42–43; recommendations on choosing, 44

U

union rules, 6
unpleasant tasks, 202

V

vacations/holidays: importance of taking, 13–14, 212–213; maximizing impact of, 214–217; private practice costs of, 13; tips on planning, 213
value-added taxes, 158
virus-detection programs, 135
voice mail checking, 203

W

waiting room, 46–47, 62–65
walking to/from work, 201, 208

walls of office, 54, 55–56
washrooms, 45, 48, 63
water cooler, 63
Wealthy Barber, The (Chilton), 160
Web browsers, 108
Web-based resources: downloadable forms/sheets, 2; providing website links to, 109–110; referral services, 85
website creation, 95–112; blogs and, 108–109; browser test, 108; contact info accessibility, 112; content ideas, 99–101; design preparation, 102–105; elements to avoid in, 106; essential reasons for, 95–96; hiring a designer for, 106–107; home page considerations, 101–102; links page resources, 109–110; navigation issues, 107–108; search engine results and, 111; site address for, 97–98
wheelchair accessibility, 45
whiteboards, 58–60, 194
white-noise generator, 55
Wilde, Oscar, 33
windows of office, 48, 56
wireless broadband, 67
women, clothing tips for, 71–72

work: eliminating commute to, 15; play/leisure added to, 205–206; preventing burnout from, 225–247; schedule flexibility for, 13–15; transitioning home from, 207–209
workers' compensation, 158
worksheets: Home-to-Work Transition, 201; Potential Referral Sources, 76, 77; Private-Practice Income: Requirements and Projections, 145; Private-Practice Task Balancing, 232; Work-to-Home Transition, 207; Your Burnout Warning Signs, 245
workshops: continuing-education, 211, 234; costs of presenting, 140–141
work-to-home transition, 207–209
writing: books, 234; schedules, 204; session notes, 197–198; task lists, 204–205

Y

yellow pages, 85

Z

zero-based budgeting, 6

more tools for your practice
from new**harbinger**publications, inc.

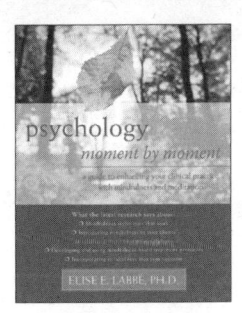

Sign up for our Book Alerts at www.newharbinger.com

PSYCHOLOGY MOMENT BY MOMENT
A Guide to Enhancing Your Clinical Practice with Mindfulness & Meditation
US $49.95 / ISBN: 978-1572248953
Also available as an **eBook** at **newharbinger.com**

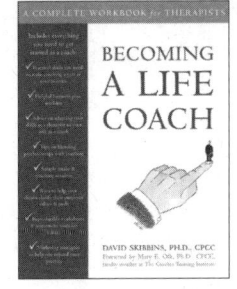

BECOMING A LIFE COACH
A Complete Workbook for Therapists
US $24.95 / ISBN: 978-1572245006

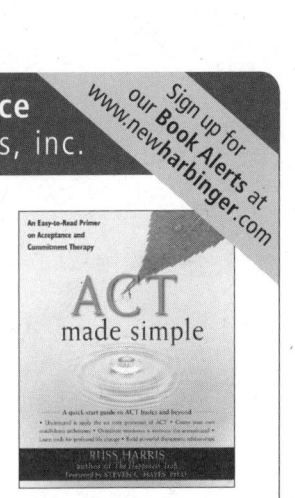

ACT MADE SIMPLE
An Easy-To-Read Primer on Acceptance & Commitment Therapy
US $39.95 / ISBN: 978-1572247055
Also available as an **eBook** at **newharbinger.com**

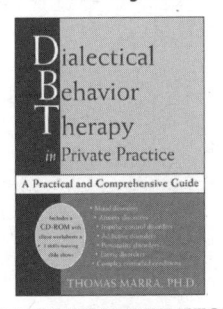

DIALECTICAL BEHAVIOR THERAPY IN PRIVATE PRACTICE
A Practical & Comprehensive Guide
US $57.95 / ISBN: 978-1572244207
Also available as an **eBook** at **newharbinger.com**

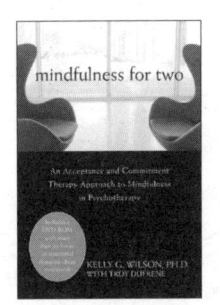

MINDFULNESS FOR TWO
An Acceptance & Commitment Therapy Approach to Mindfulness in Psychotherapy
US $49.95 / ISBN: 978-1608822669

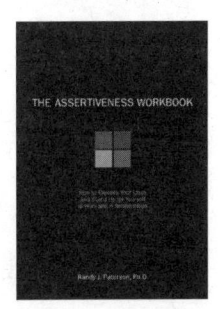

THE ASSERTIVENESS WORKBOOK
How to Express Your Ideas & Stand Up for Yourself at Work & in Relationships
US $21.95 / ISBN: 978-1572242098
Also available as an **eBook** at **newharbinger.com**

available from
new**harbinger**publications, inc.
and fine booksellers everywhere

To order, call toll free **1-800-748-6273**
or visit our online bookstore at **www.newharbinger.com**
(VISA, MC, AMEX / prices subject to change without notice)

Sign up to receive QUICK TIPS for THERAPISTS—
fast and free solutions to common client situations mental health professionals encounter. Written by New Harbinger authors, some of the most prominent names in psychology today, **QUICK TIPS for THERAPISTS** are short, helpful emails that will help enhance your client sessions. Visit www.newharbinger.com and click on "Quick Tips for Therapists" to sign up today.